Transesophageal Echocardiography

Echocardiography
Clinical and Intraoperative Applications

TRANSESOPHAGEAL ECHOCARDIOGRAPHY
Clinical and Intraoperative Applications

JOSÉ MISSRI, M.D.

Associate Professor
Department of Medicine
University of Connecticut School of Medicine
Farmington, Connecticut
Associate Medical Director
Hoffman Heart Institute of Connecticut
Director
Cardiac Catheterization Laboratory
Director
Cardiac Noninvasive Laboratory
Saint Francis Hospital and Medical Center
Hartford, Connecticut

With a contribution by
Terence Rafferty, M.D.

Associate Professor
Department of Anesthesiology
Yale University School of Medicine
Attending Anesthesiologist
Department of Anesthesiology
Yale-New Haven Hospital
New Haven, Connecticut

Churchill Livingstone
New York, Edinburgh, London, Melbourne, Tokyo

Library of Congress Cataloging-in-Publication Data

Missri, José, date
    Transesophageal echocardiography : clinical and intraoperative
applications / José Missri with a contribution by Terence Rafferty.
        p. cm.
    Includes bibliographical references and index.
    ISBN 0-443-08852-7
    1. Transesophageal echocardiography. I. Rafferty, Terence.
II. Title.
    [DNLM: 1. Echocardiography—methods. 2. Heart Diseases-
diagnosis. WG 141.5.E2 M6785t]
RC683.5.T83M57 1993
616.1'207543—dc20
DNLM/DLC
for Library of Congress   92-23799
                                                              CIP

Distributed in the United Kingdom by Churchill Livingstone, Robert Stevenson House, 1–3 Baxter's Place, Leith Walk, Edinburgh EH1 3AF, and by associated companies, branches, and representatives throughout the world.

The Publishers have made every effort to trace the copyright holders for borrowed material. If they have inadvertently overlooked any, they will be pleased to make the necessary arrangements at the first opportunity.

Acquisitions Editor: *Avé McCracken*
Copy Editor: *David Terry*
Production Designer: *Charlie Lebeda*
Production Supervisor: *Jeanine Furino*

Printed in Singapore

First published in 1993   7 6 5 4 3 2 1

To my wife, daughters, and parents

Preface

Transesophageal echocardiography (TEE) represents a major technological advance in noninvasive evaluation of cardiac patients. The standard transthoracic echocardiographic approach is frequently limited by inadequate external acoustic windows, which often occur in association with obesity, chronic obstructive pulmonary disease, thick or deformed chest walls, and chest trauma and in acutely sick patients on respirators. In these patients, TEE can provide important diagnostic information because chest wall interference and intrathoracic attenuation are eliminated. Furthermore, the close proximity of the heart and thoracic aorta to the echocardiographic transducer allows the use of high-frequency transesophageal transducers (5 MHz), which also have both color and conventional Doppler capability and provide high-resolution images of the cardiac structures that are consistently superior in quality to those obtained using the transthoracic approach. More recently, two transducers have been mounted sequentially on the tip of the transesophageal echocardiographic probe, which allows use of biplane imaging to visualize cardiac structures in orthogonal planes.

Transesophageal Echocardiography provides the cardiologist, cardiac surgeon, echocardiographic technologist, and anesthesiologist with an extensive, in-depth, and up-to-date reference on the current indications, values, and limitations of TEE when used in conjunction with the standard, transthoracic, two-dimensional echocardiographic Doppler examination. The book takes the format of an atlas-text, extensively illustrated with schematic line drawings and two-dimensional color flow images.

Although the introduction of single-plane transesophageal imaging was an important advance, providing for consistently high-quality images, one drawback has been the method's inability to provide orthogonal tomographic views. The advent of the biplane transesophageal probe, which can image in both transverse and longitudinal planes, is an important recent advance. Biplanar imaging, which has become the modality of choice for transesophageal ultrasound imaging of the heart, is utilized throughout the text, with emphasis on cases in which biplane TEE has permitted more confident diagnosis.

The book is organized into various chapters that provide the reader with standards for setting up a well-equipped TEE laboratory and for performing a comprehensive biplane examination. Detailed reviews of biplane tomographic anatomy of the heart and aorta and descriptions of the various clinical applications and limitations of TEE are provided. There are specific chapters on the assessment of aortic and mitral valve diseases, prosthetic valve function, endocarditis, intracardiac masses, imaging of coronary arteries, congenital heart disease in the adult, and the evaluation of the source of embolization. The utility of TEE in suspected aortic dissection and in the evaluation of critically ill patients in the intensive care unit is thoroughly discussed. There are specific chapters dealing with the importance of intraoperative TEE in assessing surgical repair of valvular heart disease, correction of congenital anomalies, and monitoring of myocardial ischemia and cardiac function in high-risk patients with heart disease.

I am grateful to Dr. Terry Rafferty for contributing Chapter 17, "Intraoperative Monitoring of Ischemia and Systolic Cardiac Function." His extensive experience as an anesthesiologist using TEE provides the reader with a different approach to intraoperative TEE and complements the rest of the text.

The Echocardiography Laboratory at the Hoffman Heart Institute of Connecticut, Saint Francis Hospital and Medical Center serves as a major referral for transthoracic and transesophageal Doppler echocardiographic studies. We have been fortunate in acquiring state-of-the-art technology that has made this book possible. We are committed to providing our patients with the best available noninvasive technology, training future cardiologists, and providing preceptorship training in TEE to practicing cardiologists. *Transesophageal Echocardiography* represents our desire to foster this exciting and emerging field of cardiac evaluation.

José Missri, M.D.

Acknowledgments

The preparation and completion of this book would not have been possible without the contributions of a number of individuals who gave their time and talent. I am grateful to Donna Crowal for her hard work in the preparation of the manuscript, to Joseph Milhomens and Dan Aitchison for the photography, and to Christopher Roy of Biomedical Communications at the University of Connecticut Health Center for the artwork.

Special thanks is accorded to Daniel Goodfield, chief echocardiography sonographer, who has made it possible to run a high-quality echocardiography laboratory and whose expertise I have counted on in producing this book. I am indebted to Dr. Rami Gal, of the University of Wisconsin Medical School in Milwaukee, who so kindly permitted me to use material from his laboratory relating to malignant cardiac tumors, mitral valvuloplasty, and congenital ventricular septal defect.

It is a personal pleasure to be associated with Dr. Robert Jeresaty, Medical Director of the Hoffman Heart Institute, Dr. David D'Eramo, President and Chief Executive Officer of Saint Francis Hospital, Dr. J. David Schnatz, Chairman of the Department of Medicine, Saint Francis Hospital, and Dr. Edward Johnson, Vice President, Saint Francis Hospital. They are committed to high-quality patient care, education, and research.

I wish to express my gratitude to my colleagues at Saint Francis Hospital and at other medical institutions, who permitted me to draw upon their experience and material. Our medical students, residents, and cardiology fellows provide the interest and stimulation for my role as clinician and teacher. It is always a pleasure to work alongside Churchill Livingstone and in particular Avé McCracken, Executive Editor, and David Terry, copy editor. Their advice and assistance is greatly appreciated. Finally, I want to express my deep appreciation to my family for their interest and encouragement.

Contents

1 Historical Perspective

Transesophageal echocardiography (TEE) is a new and rapidly expanding technicque that permits ultrasonic imaging of the cardiac structures and great vessels via the retrocardiac esophagus. Although advances in 2-D echocardiography, pulsed and continuous-wave Doppler, and color Doppler imaging have revolutionized noninvasive assessment of cardiac disorders, these modalities may be limited in many patients by several factors. These impediments include acoustic attenuation from structures in the thorax (lungs, subcutaneous tissues, and ribs) and heart (prosthetic valve construction materials and calcification of native valves). In these patients, TEE can provide important diagnostic information because chest wall interference and intrathoracic attenuation are eliminated. Furthermore, the close vicinity of the heart and thoracic aorta to the echocardiographic probe permits the use of higher-frequency, near-focus transducers, which produce better resolution and an improved signal-to-noise ratio. In addition, some structures that are poorly visualized by standard transthoracic echocardiography (TTE) are better observed by the transesophageal approach, including wide areas of both atrial chambers, prosthetic valves, proximal coronary arteries, and the thoracic aorta. Commercially available TEE probes, capable of 2-D imaging, real-time color Doppler imaging, pulsed and continuous-wave Doppler interrogation have been incorporated into small flexible gastroscope devices to permit easy and safe esophageal introduction in both awake and anesthetized patients.

HISTORICAL DEVELOPMENT OF TEE

In 1968 a new generation of gastroscopes with a steerable tip became available. This led to the first cardiac investigation with ultrasound via the esophagus[1] (Table 1-1). Side and Goslin used a dual-element construction mounted on a standard gastroscope to obtain continuous-wave Doppler recordings of cardiac flow. The use of Doppler recording through the esophagus was further expanded with the use of pulsed Doppler with a single element. In 1976, Frazin and associates[2] attached a single-crystal M-mode ultrasound transducer to the tip of a cable (Fig. 1-1) and studied the feasibility of obtaining accurate measurements of the aortic root and mitral valve motion in awake patients. However, they failed to visualize the

Table 1-1. Historical Development of Transesophageal Echocardiography[a]

1976	M-mode TEE
1981	Two-dimensional TEE (3.5-mHz transducer mounted on modified gastroscope)

Pathway of Development	
U.S.	Europe
Japan	Japan

Intraoperative monitoring of left ventricular function
Ambulatory diagnostic

1987	Color Doppler (5.0-mHz probe)
1989	Biplane TEE and uniplane pediatric TEE
1992	Development of multiplanar TEE tissue characterization

[a]See text for details.

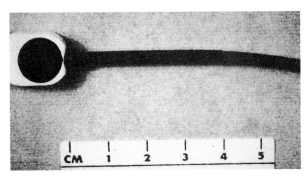

Fig. 1-1. Esophageal 3.5-MHz nonfocused M-mode transducer developed by Frazin. (From Frazin et al.,[2] with permission.)

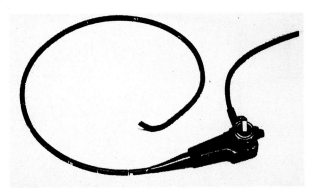

Fig. 1-2. Hanrath's modified gastroscope with phased-array transducer fixed at the flexible tip. (From Schlüter et al.,[6] with permission.)

left ventricle due to limited position of the transesophageal probe. In 1977, Matsuzaki and associates[3] attached a 3-MHz 6-mm transducer to the tip of a gastro-camera and obtained left ventricular images, which were used to evaluate left ventricular anterolateral wall motion in awake patients with coronary artery disease.

Hanrath et al.[4] were the first to modify a gastroscope and mount a 2-D phased-array ultrasound transducer to obtain the first 2-D echocardiograms from the esophagus (Fig. 1-2). This device showed promise as a means of imaging the heart and thoracic aorta. Initial studies[4-6] and anatomic correlations[7-9] aroused interest in its clinical values. Clinical applications for this technique, both in surgical and in outpatient settings, were studied extensively by Hanrath in Germany.[4,5] Intraoperative monitoring of global and regional myocardial function[10,11] and recognition of intracavitary air during neurosurgical procedures with patients in the upright position[12] were two of the initial clinical applications of TEE between 1982 and 1986.

In the United States between 1982 and 1986, the use of this technique was limited only to certain institutions for assessment of intraoperative left ventricular function and myocardial ischemia in high-risk noncardiac surgical patients.[13,14] During this time, however, investigators primarily in Europe and Japan explored various applications of 2-D TEE outside the operating room. In the United States, more widespread application of this technique did not occur

until 1987 and 1988, when a high-resolution 64-element transesophageal probe with pulsed Doppler and color Doppler imaging capabilities became available. In 1989, Omoto et al.[15-16] developed biplane adult and uniplane pediatric transesophageal echo probes. Ritter and Thys[17] recently reviewed their experience with a prototype pediatric probe. This led to an explosive and worldwide application of TEE that broke down previous perceptions of echocardiography as only a noninvasive technique and established the era of "invasive echocardiography." Thus, TEE is now extensively applied, both in ambulatory and in operative patients, by cardiologists as well as anesthesiologists.

Transesophageal echo-anatomic correlations were reported initially by Schlüter et al.[6] during the early 1980s and in more detail by Seward et al.[18] for single-plane imaging in 1988 and for biplane imaging in 1990.[19]

REFERENCES

1. Side CD, Goslin RG. Non-surgical assessment of cardiac function. Nature 1971; 232:335–336.
2. Frazin L, Talano JV, Stephanides L, et al. Esophageal echocardiography. Circulation 1976; 54:102–108.
3. Matsuzaki M, Ikee Y, Maeda S, et al. A clinical application and technique of esophageal echocardiography (abst). Jpn Circ J 1977; 41:772.
4. Hanrath P, Kremer P, Langenstein BA, et al. Transösophageale Echokardiographie: Ein neues Verfahren zur dynamischen Ventrikelfunktions-analyse. Dtsch Med Wochenschr 1981; 106:523–525.
5. Souquet J, Hanrath P, Zitelli, et al. Transesophageal phased array for imaging the heart. IEEE Trans Biomed Eng 1982; 29:707–712.

6. Schlüter M, Langenstein BA, Polster J, et al. Transesophageal cross-sectional echocardiography with a phased array transducer system: technique and initial clinical results. Br Heart J 1982; 48:67–72.

7. Schlüter M, Hinrich A, Thier W, et al. Transesophageal two-dimensional echocardiography: comparison of ultrasonic and anatomic sections. Am J Cardiol 1984; 53:1173–1178.

8. Toma Y, Matsuda Y, Matsuzaki M, et al. Determination of atrial size by esophageal echocardiography. Am J Cardiol 1983; 52:878–880.

9. Seward JB, Tajik AJ, DiMagno EP. Esophageal phased-array sector echocardiography: an anatomic study. In Hanrath P, Bleifeld W, Souquet J, (eds): Cardiovascular Diagnosis by Ultrasound: Transesophageal, Computerized, Contrast, Doppler Echocardiography. The Hague: Martinus Nijhoff, 1982, pp 270–279.

10. Schiller NB. Evaluation of cardiac function during surgery by transesophageal 2-dimensional echocardiography. In Hanrath P, Bliefeld W, Souquet J (eds): Cardiovascular Diagnosis by Ultrasound: Transesophageal, Computerized, Contrast, Doppler Echocardiography. The Hague: Martinus Nijhoff, 1982, pp 289–293.

11. Kremer P, Schwartz L, Cahalan MK, et al. Intraoperative monitoring of left ventricular performance by transesophageal m-mode and 2-D echocardiography (abst). Am J Cardiol 1982; 49:956.

12. Cucchiara RF, Nugent M, Seward JB, Messick JM. Air embolism in upright neurosurgical patients: detection and localization by two-dimensional transesophageal echocardiography. Anesthesiology 1984; 60:353–355.

13. Smith JS. Intraoperative detection of myocardial ischemia in high-risk patients: electrocardiography versus two-dimensional transesophageal echocardiography. Circulation 1985; 72:1015–1019.

14. Roizen MF, Beaupre PN, Alpert RA, et al. Monitoring with two-dimensional transesophageal echocardiography: comparison of myocardial function in patients undergoing supraceliac, suprarenal-infraceliac, or infrarenal aortic occlusion. J Vasc Surg 1984; 1:300–303.

15. Omoto R, Kyo S, Matsumara M, et al. Biplane color transesophageal Doppler echocardiography (color TEE): its advantages and limitations. Int J Cardiol Imag 1989; 4:57–58.

16. Omoto R, Kyo S, Matsumard M, et al. Biplane color Doppler transesophageal echocardiography: its impact on cardiovascular surgery and further technological progress in the probe, a matrix phased-array biplane probe. Echocardiography 1989; 423–430.

17. Ritter SB, Thys D. Pediatric transesophageal color flow imaging: smaller probes for smaller hearts. Echocardiography 1989; 6:431–440.

18. Seward JB, Khandheria BK, Oh JK, et al. Transesophageal echocardiography: technique, anatomic correlations, implementation and clinical applications. Mayo Clin Proc 1988; 63:649–680.

19. Seward JB, Khandheria BK, Edwards WD, et al. Biplanar transesophageal echocardiography: anatomic correlations, image orientation, and clinical applications. Mayo Clin Proc 1990; 65:1193–1213.

2 Equipment and Laboratory Setup

TEE EQUIPMENT AND CURRENT PROBE TECHNOLOGY

TEE imaging is usually performed using phased-array transducers (5.0 MHz, 48 to 64 elements) incorporated into a modified flexible endoscope without fiberoptics (9- to 11-mm shaft) interfaced to standard echocardiographic machines, providing combined 2-D, pulsed, and continuous-wave Doppler and color Doppler imaging (Figs. 2-1 and 2-2). Control knobs at the base of the endoscope permit flexion of the tip in anteroposterior as well as left and right lateral directions, enabling optimization of image quality and orientation (Fig. 2-3). Current probe technology incorporates thermistors into the tip to monitor probe temperatures and automatically shut down when temperatures exceed 42 °C. This safeguard is required because malfunctioning ultrasonic crystals can convert electrical energy into heat rather than ultrasound. This safety feature may terminate examinations of febrile patients or of patients being weaned from extracorporeal bypass in whom warm blood returning from the pump to the aorta locally heats the heart. Although we are not currently experiencing this problem, many manufacturers are developing manual override features for these thermistor circuits. A second safety feature is electrical testing circuits for current leakage; these are periodically employed to protect the patient from the remote possibility of electrical shock.

Most manufacturers of single-plane probes mounted the transducer in such a way to allow a 90-degree horizontal or transverse tomographic plane of section. The tip has 90 degrees or more of forward and reverse mobility and approximately 70 degrees of lateral mobility. Hewlett-Packard Company (Andover, MA) manufactures a transesophageal probe with 64 phased-array imaging crystals, incorporated into the tip of a flexible gastroscope-like device (no fiberoptics or suction capabilities) with a carrier frequency of 5.0 MHz. This probe is 100 cm long and has a shaft diameter of 10 mm, a tip width of 14 mm, and a tip length of 27 mm.

The recently introduced Hewlett-Packard biplane transesophageal imaging transducer has a carrier frequency of 5.0 MHz with two 48-element array imaging transducers for biplane transesophageal imaging. Two perpendicular scanning planes — transverse (horizontal) and longitudinal (vertical) — permit imaging of two separate (not simultaneous) cross sections of the heart. The distal transducer provides a transverse plane of section and a more proximal transducer permits sectioning in a longitudinal plane (Fig. 2-4). The probe has capabilities for pulsed, continuous-wave and color Doppler imaging.

Aloka (Tokyo) and Corometrics (Wallingford, CT) manufacture uniplane and biplane adult and uniplane pediatric transesophageal probes interphased with the Aloka phased-array color Doppler echocardiographic imaging system. The single-plane adult probe employs a 48-element, horizontal or transverse plane, scanning phase-array transducer operating at a frequency of 5.0 MHz. The biplane probe contains two transducers, each containing 32 elements and

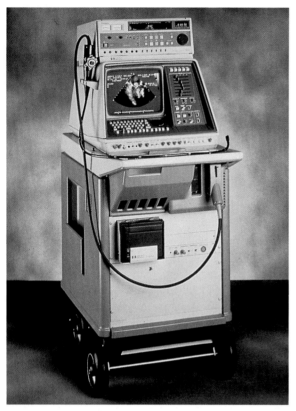

Fig. 2-1. Hewlett-Packard ultrasound imaging system with transesophageal probe capable of performing 2-D imaging, Doppler, and color Doppler mapping.

operating at a frequency of 5.0 MHz. The pediatric probe, also manufactured by Aloka Corporation, has a transducer containing 24 elements and operating at a frequency of 5.0 MHz. The length of the pediatric echoscope is 70 to 100 cm and has a shaft diameter of 6.8 mm, a maximum tip width of 7 mm, and a tip length of 14 mm.

Other manufacturers of transesophageal probes include Acuson Corporation (Mountain View, CA), which manufactures a transesophageal probe with 64 elements that operates at a frequency of 5.0 MHz. General Electric Medical Systems (Milwaukee, WI) offers a single-plane probe with a 64-element transducer and a biplane probe with two 64-element transducers. This probe has a capability of performing both pulsed and continuous-wave Doppler. Toshiba Corporation (Japan) and Diasonics (Palo Alto, CA) supply a transesophageal echo probe with 64 elements that operates at a frequency of 5.0 MHz. Advanced Technology Laboratories (ATL, Bellevue, WA) makes a TEE probe similar in design to the other probes.

LABORATORY SETUP

The performance of a safe and successful outpatient transesophageal examination is dependent on a well-

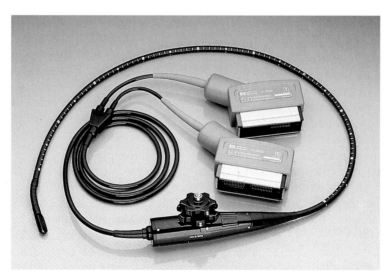

Fig. 2-2. A 5.0-MHz phased-array imaging transducer with two 48-element arrays for biplane transesophageal imaging. Two rotary knobs located at the base handle control the mobility of the tip.

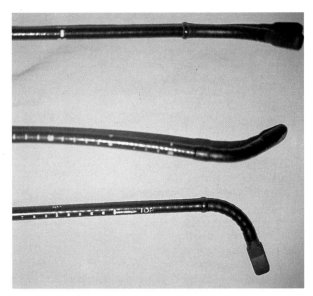

Fig. 2-3. Manipulations of transesophageal endoscope. The tip of the scope provides 90 degrees of forward (anteflexion) and reverse (retroflexion) and approximately 70 degrees of lateral mobility. The tip of scope can also be advanced, withdrawn, and rotated leftward or rightward.

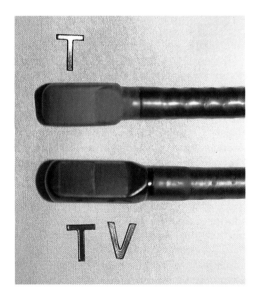

Fig. 2-4. Configuration of the uniplane and biplane transesophageal transducer. The uniplane transducer provides images in transverse plane (T), and the biplane transducer provides images in transverse (T) and longitudinal or vertical (V) planes. The centers of the two arrays are separated by 1.0 cm (Hewlett-Packard transducers).

equipped TEE laboratory as well as patient education and preparation before examination. TEE should be performed by a physician who is well trained in echocardiography, including standard 2-D and Doppler techniques, and who is very familiar with tomographic cardiac anatomy. In addition, it is mandatory that the physician be trained in passing an endoscope; the training should be given by either a gastroenterologist skilled in upper gastrointestinal (GI) endoscopy or another cardiologist experienced in TEE (see Ch. 3 for training requirements).

The cardiologist should be assisted by a cardiac sonographer, whose important roles include the following: (1) ensuring that the transesophageal echo room is equipped with the necessary supplies; (2) setting up the equipment and providing technical help in adjusting the machine during the examination; (3) helping in patient education and preparation; (4) monitoring heart rate, blood pressure, respiration, and oxygen saturation before and during the examination; and (5) cleaning, disinfecting, and storing the esophageal probe following the procedure.

The TEE laboratory should be set up somewhat similarly to the endoscopy room (Table 2-1). It should be equipped with cardiopulmonary resuscitation equip-

Table 2-1. Requirements for Equipment and Supplies in the TEE Laboratory

Laboratory equipment
    Cardiopulmonary resuscitation equipment
    Oxygen and suction capabilities
    Pulse oximeter
    Blood pressure monitoring
    Electrocardiographic monitoring
Supplies
    Gloves
    Disposable towels
    Tongue depressors
    Bite guard and emesis basin
    Intravenous access (angiocath or butterfly needle)
    Heparin lock flush solution
    Sterile normal saline solution and three-way stopcocks for contrast study
Cleaning and protection of probe
    2% glutaraldehyde solution (Cidex, Metricide)
    Wash basin
    Mounted wall rack (Fig. 2-5)
    Carrying case

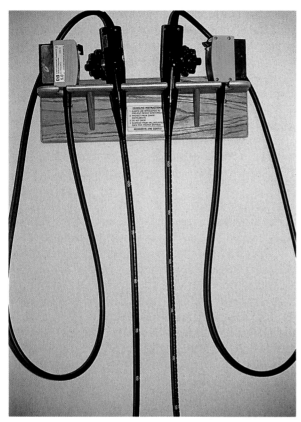

Fig. 2-5. Mounted wall rack used for storage of esophageal probes.

Table 2-2. Medications Used in the TEE Laboratory

Oropharyngeal topical anesthetic agents
    10% lydocaine oral spray (Xylocaine)
    20% benzocaine (Hurricaine)
    14% benzocaine (Cetacaine)

Sedation[a]
    Midazolam
    Diazepam
    Lorazepam
    Meperidine

Mucosal drying agents[a,b]
    Glycopyrrolate

Prophylaxis for endocarditis
    As per recommendations of the American Heart Association
    for high-risk patients

Emergency cardiac medications[a]
    Intravenous atropine
    Intravenous propranolol, verapamil, or adenosine
    Lidocaine hydrochloride
    Diphenhydramine hydrochloride injection
    Epinephrine injection

[a] The package insert for each drug should be consulted for use and dosage as approved by the FDA.
[b] Use varies.

ment, oxygen and suction capabilities, pulse oximeter, blood pressure, and electrocardiographic monitoring. A wash basin is necessary for cleaning the transesophageal echoscope after each examination.

Other necessary supplies include disposable gloves and towels, tongue depressors, a bite guard, and intravenous access needles or angiocath. We routinely perform echo contrast studies with agitated saline, but other contrast agents (e.g., indocyanine green dye, albumin aggregates, or polysaccharide microspheres) can be used.

Ambulatory TEE protocol is based on the standard for upper gastroenterologic endoscopy in cardiac patients. A medication closet should be located inside the laboratory, in which the necessary medications can be stored (Table 2-2). These include the following:

Oropharyngeal topical anesthesia. Serial applications of 10 percent lidocaine spray initially to the back of the tongue and posterior pharyngeal wall will suppress the gag reflex (Fig. 2-6). It is best accomplished by progressively deeper applications, testing the gag reflex to titrate the number of applications needed. Those with a pronounced gag reflex and difficulty in having the oropharynx sprayed will require sedation. Other topical anesthetic agents include 20 percent benzocaine or 14 percent benzocaine preparations.

Sedation. The need for sedation is variable but is highly recommended in patients who have (1) anxiety; (2) suspected aortic dissection; and (3) the potential need for serial TEE studies (e.g., those having infective endocarditis, aortic dissection, and prosthetic valves). Above all, it is useful when the physician is in an early phase of training and needs additional time to obtain and recognize the tomographic anatomy. Sedation can be accomplished using midazolam hydrochloride 0.5 to 2 mg administered slowly, or meperidine hydrochloride 12.5 to 25 mg IV.

Mucosal drying agents. Some laboratories advocate the use of a mucosal drying agent (glycopyrrolate) to prevent excessive oral secretions. However, the advantage of this

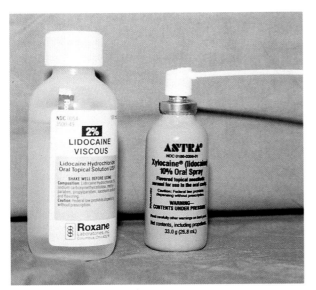

Fig. 2-6. Lidocaine spray *(right)* used for oropharyngeal topical anesthesia and viscous lidocaine *(left)* used to lubricate the flexible tip of the esophageal probe. The long probe on the lidocaine spray is used for spraying deep in the oropharynx.

effect is outweighed by the associated high frequency of sore throats following the procedure.[1] Low-pressure wall suction with a dental sucker controls secretions without the side effects of an anticholinergic drug.

Prophylaxis for endocarditis. The use of antibiotic prophylaxis for TEE is controversial, without definitive studies as a guideline. We recommend antibiotic prophylaxis for high-risk patients (i.e., those with prosthetic valves and a prior history of endocarditis), according to the recommendations of the American Heart Association for upper endoscopy (see Ch. 3).

Emergency cardiac medications. Such medications include (1) atropine for emergency use in bradyarrhythmias; (2) intravenous propranolol, verapamil, or adenosine for emergency use in rapid supraventricular arrhythmias; (3) lidocaine hydrochloride for emergency use for ventricular arrhythmias; and (4) diphenhydramine hydrochloride injection and epinephrine injection for emergency use in hypersensitive or anaphylactic reactions.

REFERENCE

1. Khandheria BK. Safety of transesophageal echocardiography in awake patients: experience with 400 procedures. J Am Coll Cardiol 1989; 13:225A (abst).

3 Techniques, Indications, Complications, and Training Requirements

PREPARATION FOR THE EXAMINATION

The patient should abstain from oral intake for at least 4 to 6 hours before the procedure. In emergencies, the examination can be performed without fasting, such as in patients with aortic dissection. The patient should be informed of the potential risks of the procedure and the specific reason for performing the TEE examination and an informed consent obtained. The patient's history should be reviewed for possible contraindications to esophageal intubation, including a history of dysphagia or esophageal disease, mediastinal radiation, recent gastroesophageal surgery, and active upper gastrointestinal bleeding (Table 3-1). A drug and allergy history also must be obtained. If there is a history of esophageal pathology, a gastroenterologic consultation and endoscopy should be performed prior to TEE.

Dentures and oral prosthesis are removed before the examination. An intravenous (IV) line is established; monitoring of the patient's vital signs, including heart rate, blood pressure, respiration, and color, is initiated prior to the examination. A pulse oximeter is recommended particularly for those patients receiving intravenous sedation. Topical oropharyngeal anesthesia is achieved with serial applications of a local anesthetic aerosol spray solution, initially to the back of the tongue and posterior pharyngeal wall to suppress the gag reflex. It is best accomplished with progressively deeper applications, testing the gag reflex to titrate the number of applications needed. Those with a very pronounced gag reflex and difficulty

having the oropharynx sprayed will require more sedation.

We routinely do not use sedation. In anxious and awake patients, however, our drug of choice is midazolam hydrochloride in a dose of 0.5 to 3 mg IV, over a period of 1 to 2 minutes. The dose is reduced in elderly or debilitated patients. This drug dispels anxiety, produces sedation, and provides amnesia. Close monitoring of the patient's color, respiration, blood pressure, and oxygen saturation by pulse oximetry is important in patients with conscious sedation. Elderly patients have a less sensitive gag reflex and tolerate the procedure much better than do younger patients. Other agents that might be used include diazepam, meperidine, and other similar compounds.

The use of a drying agent is controversial, and we have never used it. Some laboratories administer an intravenous bolus of 0.2 mg of glycopyrrolate (Robinul). This anticholinergic agent may produce a mild increase in heart rate in patients with high resting vagal tone or atrial fibrillation. It may also cause temporary blurring of vision as well as drowsiness. This agent should not be employed in patients with a history of glaucoma, bronchospasm, or urinary retention or in patients who have resting tachycardia.

The value of prophylaxis against endocarditis is controversial. A recent study from the Mayo Clinic found no significant bacteremia attributable to pathogenic oroflora during TEE.[1] In another study,[2] multiple

Table 3-1. Relative Contraindications to TEE

Uncooperative patient

History
    Dysphagia
    Mediastinal radiation
    Active upper gastrointestinal bleeding
    Penetrating or blunt chest trauma
    Recent gastroesophageal surgery

Esophageal pathology
    Strictures
    Diverticulum
    Varices
    Fistulas
    Esophagitis
    Scleroderma
    Bleeding disorders
    Carcinoma

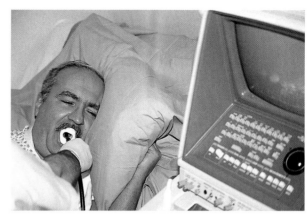

Fig. 3-1. Esophageal intubation of conscious patient. The patient is positioned in the left decubitus position with the head flexed. A bite guard is used, and oral suctioning is placed next to patient.

blood cultures in 83 patients undergoing TEE did not find evidence of bacteremia in even a single case. These data show that the risk of bacteremia and possible endocarditis is low with only esophageal intubation. At our institution, we do not routinely administer antibiotic prophylaxis except in patients with prosthetic heart valves or a history of previous endocarditis. In more than 600 cases where antibiotic prophylaxis was not routinely used prior to TEE, we have not been aware of any cases of endocarditis. In order to avoid masking the presence of suspected organisms in blood cultures, patients undergoing TEE as part of an evaluation for infective endocarditis are not given endocarditis prophylaxis.

TECHNIQUE OF PROBE INSERTION

The probe should be inspected carefully for flaws, bite marks, and discontinuity that may cause electrical leakage. The probe controls should be manipulated to ensure normal function. The probe is always introduced with the controls unlocked and in the neutral position.

Conscious Patients

Introduction of the esophageal probe is normally done with the patient in the left lateral decubitus position, with the neck flexed until the chin rests on

the chest to facilitate easy passage of the probe (Fig. 3-1). Because of the risk of aspiration, endoscopy with the patient in a supine position is not recommended. The probe is well lubricated with surgical or lidocaine jelly to the 15-cm mark and is slightly flexed before the procedure to ensure easy passage into the esophagus. Both the operator and the assistant should wear disposable gloves. A bite guard is not required in edentulous patients but should be used in all other patients, to avoid accidental biting and damage to the echoscope (Fig. 3-2). We routinely insert the left index finger into the patient's mouth and advance it to the posterior aspect of the tongue. With adequate local anesthesia, the patient will not gag. With the left index finger at the base of the tongue,

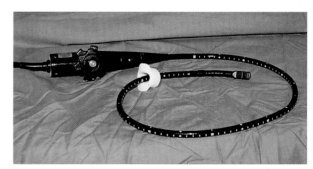

Fig. 3-2. Biplane transesophageal probe fitted with disposable bite guard.

the tip of the partially flexed transducer is advanced into the mouth with the right hand. The tip of the endoscope is passed beneath the left index finger. Gentle downward pressure on the distal part of the endoscope will direct the tip of the transducer toward the esophageal orifice. Reflexes will draw the larynx upward and the epiglottis posteriorly; thereby preventing entry into the trachea. With the tip of the endoscope at the esophageal orifice, the patient is requested to swallow. This action will direct the scope into the upper part of the esophagus. The endoscope is firmly advanced but should not be forced. If resistance is encountered, the endoscope should be redirected. The patient's gag reflex is heightened as long as the tip of the endoscope remains above the tracheal carina (20 to 25 cm from the incisors). Thus, initial advancement of the instrument to approximately 25 cm into the esophagus is essential. After introduction of the probe, the bite guard is introduced over the patient's teeth to protect both the probe and the patient's oropharynx.

Another alternative is to place the bite guard between the patient's teeth, and the tube is advanced to the opening of the bite guard as the patient swallows. This technique is safer, both for the operator's finger and for the probe. It may be necessary in some instances, however, to use the left index finger to direct the probe, if resistance is met.

During a routine procedure, the heart rate and blood pressure commonly increase slightly, but this is generally transient and lasts only a few minutes. During the examination, the patient might feel nauseated or begin to gag. Cessation of manipulation of the probes often makes the patient more comfortable, permitting the examination to continue. Nausea and vomiting generally occur when the probe is in the stomach, and the probe may have to be withdrawn into the esophagus. Routine intermittent suctioning of oral and pharyngeal secretions is performed in all patients, to prevent aspiration. It is important to warn the patient not to swallow secretions after the probe has been inserted and to signal if he or she requires oral suctioning. Occasionally, the patient may vomit during the procedure. This generally occurs in patients who have ingested food or liquid before the procedure. The TEE examination is generally completed within 10 to 15 minutes.

Conscious Patients with Endotracheal Tube

In a conscious patient who is in an intensive care unit (ICU), with an endotracheal tube in place and on a respirator, intravenous sedation and analgesia are usually required prior to esophageal intubation. Occasionally, intravenous pancuronium bromide (Pavulone) is required to induce relaxation of the skeletal muscles of the jaw and neck to facilitate insertion of the echo probe. This drug sometimes causes tachycardia and hypertension, which should be monitored.

Unconscious Patients

Introduction of the transesophageal probe in the anesthetized or unconscious patient in the operating room or in an ICU is technically easier than in the conscious patient because of the absence of gagging, retching, or coughing. The patient is usually recumbent and need not be in the left decubitus position if intubated. The head should be in the midline position with the neck slightly flexed. The endotracheal tube should be positioned to one side of the mouth, to provide sufficient room for the transesophageal echocardiographic probe. Catheters within the esophagus (e.g., a nasal gastric tube, feeding tube, or temperature probe) are often removed to avoid potential kinking, knotting, or intertwining of two devices. The presence of a second catheter in the esophagus may interfere with satisfactory acquisition of images.

The flexible tip of the echoscope is lubricated with surgical or lidocaine jelly and is blindly introduced by directing the tube in the midline into the posterior part of the pharynx. Digital guidance or visualization of the posterior pharynx with a laryngoscope is occasionally necessary to guide probe placement into the esophagus. Other maneuvers that can facilitate esophagoscopy include manual lifting of the laryngeal cartilage forward with additional neck flexion and temporary deflation of the cuff of the endotracheal tube.

Postprocedure Precautions

If any of the sedatives are used, it is essential that the patient be observed for approximately 30 minutes after the procedure. Patients must be cautioned against performing tasks such as driving an automobile or operating moving machinery for 12 to 24 hours after the procedure. The patient should not take anything by mouth for 45 to 60 minutes after the procedure because the topical pharyngeal anesthesia impairs swallowing and increases the risk of aspiration.

CLEANING THE ESOPHAGEAL PROBE

The echoscope should be cleaned and inspected before and after each TEE examination. The probe should be inspected for cracks or tears in the outer casing that would prevent proper cleaning and increase the possibility of electrical hazard. After each use, the endoscope should be washed with soap or enzymatic solution (Protozyme) to remove adherent saliva and then soaked in a disinfecting solution of 2 percent glutaraldehyde (Cidex, Metricide) for at least 15 minutes (Fig. 3-3). This process will destroy any bacterial and viral contaminants. After sufficient soaking, the endoscope is washed with tap water and dried before storage.

INDICATIONS AND CURRENT APPLICATIONS

In our laboratory, requests for TEE have fallen into the following categories: suspected aortic dissection, evaluation of intracardiac thrombi and other sources of embolic episodes, dysfunction of the mitral valve prosthesis, evaluation of mitral regurgitation and adequacy of surgical repair of the mitral valve, and anatomic assessment of endocarditis and its complications and evaluation of intracardiac shunts (Tables 3-2 and 3-3) and (Fig. 3-4). In most cases, the TEE examination is best used in conjunction with the standard transthoracic echocardiographic (TTE) examination. Our data indicate that approximately 5 to 10 percent of cases referred for echocardiography TEE are indicated to enhance the limited diagnostic capability of transthoracic studies.

In our own initial experience, biplane imaging generally gave new and specific information in the following areas:

1. Aortic regurgitation severity assessment
2. Determination of the site of periprosthetic mitral regurgitation
3. More accurate assessment of the severity of mitral re-

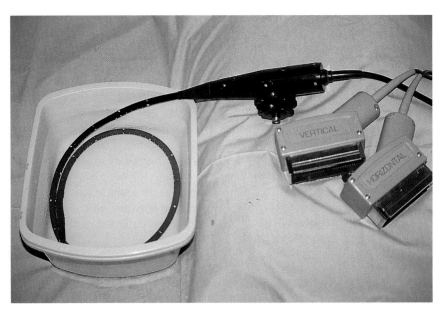

Fig. 3-3. Transesophageal probe in basin containing a disinfecting solution (Cidex).

Table 3-2. Indications for Awake/Ambulatory TEE

1. Aortic dissection/aneurysms
2. Prosthetic dysfunction
   Detection and quantitation of regurgitation
   Central vs. paravalvular regurgitation
   Endocarditis (abscesses, vegetations)
3. Intracardiac sources of emboli (thrombi)
4. Intracardiac masses (tumors)
5. Infective endocarditis (inadequate conventional echocardiography and strong suspiciion for endocarditis); abscesses
6. Valvular regurgitation (inadequate conventional echocardiography)
7. Congenital heart disease (atrial/ventricular septal defect)
8. Complications of myocardial infarction
   Ventricular septal rupture
   Papillary muscle rupture
9. Inadequate transthoracic echocardiography (essential for management)

Table 3-3. Indications for Intraoperative TEE

1. Adequacy of valvuloplasty procedures
   Mitral/tricuspid valve repair
   Mitral commissurotomy
2. Congenital heart disease: adequacy of closure of atrial/ventricular septal defect
3. Assessment of left ventricular function (selected patients)
   Global performance (contractility)
   Segmental ischemia
4. Evaluation of myotomy-myectomy in hypertrophic obstructive cardiomyopathy
5. Retained intracardiac air during cardiopulmonary bypass

gurgitation and morphologic abnormalities of the mitral valve apparatus and evaluation of mitral valve repair
4. Evaluation of regional wall motion abnormalities
5. Visualization of the ascending and descending thoracic aorta, providing for better conceptualization of any aortic disease
6. Visualization of the left atrial appendage
7. Visualization of the right ventricular outflow tract and pulmonary artery
8. Congenital heart disease, interatrial septum, and anomalous venous connection

SAFETY AND COMPLICATIONS

In experienced hands, TEE can be performed safely with almost nonexistent complications (Table 3-4). Esophageal perforation is the greatest concern and is confined to patients in whom introduction of the endoscope is difficult. The endoscopy literature reports the incidence of perforation associated with flexible esophagoscopy alone ranges from 0.02 to 0.03 percent.[3] A multicenter survey[4] of more than 10,000 examinations found a mortality rate of 0.0098 percent. This resulted from bleeding complications from a malignant lung tumor with esophageal infiltration. Unsuccessful intubation occurred in 1.9 percent because of a lack of either patient cooperation or operator experience, or both. Other complications reported

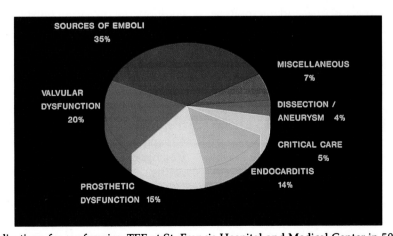

Fig. 3-4. Indications for performing TEE at St. Francis Hospital and Medical Center in 500 patients.

Table 3-4. Potential Complications of Transesophageal Echocardiography

Arrhythmias	Parotid swelling
Supraventricular tachycardia	Asthma attack
Ventricular tachycardia	Hypotension
Vasovagal reactions	Hypertension
Minor pharyngeal bleeding	Laryngospasm
Hypoxemia	Congestive heart failure
Aspiration	Hematemesis
Transient laryngeal nerve paralysis	Esophageal perforation

include vomiting, bronchial spasm, transient tachyarrhythmias, high-grade AV block, and pharyngeal bleeding.

The experience at the Mayo Clinic[5] with 1,110 patients indicated an incidence of ventricular arrhythmias in 0.3 percent, supraventricular arrhythmias in 0.3 percent, congestive heart failure in 0.2 percent, laryngeal spasm in 0.2 percent, parotid swelling in less than 0.1 percent, and unsuccessful intubation in 1.1 percent.

The effects of prolonged TEE imaging and probe manipulation on the esophagus have been studied in monkeys and mongrel dogs.[6] Dogs were studied during right heart bypass with full heparinization for 6.6 ± 0.2 hours, whereas monkeys were studied for 60 to 90 minutes in the absence of cardiopulmonary bypass and anticoagulation. Immediately after completion of TEE in each case, the esophagus was entirely excised. Detailed macroscopic and microscopic examination of the esophagus revealed no significant mucosal or thermal injury. This echocardiographic–pathologic study suggests that TEE is safe for the esophageal mucosa in animals despite prolonged use and in the presence of systemic anticoagulation. Our experience in the operating room with the transesophageal probe left in place on an average of 3.5 hours was not associated with any clinical evidence of bleeding or esophageal symptoms postoperatively.

In our first 500 TEE examinations, insertion of the TEE probe was unsuccessful in five patients (1 percent) because of a lack of patient cooperation. We have noted rare episodes of unifocal ventricular premature beats and atrial premature beats. There were no instances of perforation or bleeding complications. An important caveat is that one should never attempt to introduce the probe forcibly.

Transient recurrent laryngeal nerve paralysis has been reported in two neurosurgical patients who were undergoing extended intraoperative TEE in the sitting cervical neck flexion position.[7] Because of the rare case of aspiration and respiratory depression, the operating room should be equipped with cardiopulmonary resuscitation equipment and the capability to deliver oxygen and suction. We encountered one patient with an unsuspected large hiatal hernia interposed between the heart and the esophagus, which made it difficult to obtain satisfactory images of the heart from the transesophageal approach. The large hiatal hernia was subsequently diagnosed by computed tomography (CT) scanning.

Infectious diseases, including hepatitis, acquired immunodeficiency syndrome (AIDS), and bacterial infections can conceivably be transmitted by a contaminated TEE probe. Careful attention needs to be given to proper cleaning and sterilization of TEE probes between uses.

TRAINING REQUIREMENTS FOR PERFORMING TEE

TEE should be performed by a physician who is well trained in echocardiography, including standard 2-D Doppler and color Doppler techniques, and who is very familiar with tomographic cardiac anatomy. In addition, the physician must be trained in passing an endoscope, by either a gastroenterologist skilled in upper gastrointestinal (GI) endoscopy or by another cardiologist experienced in TEE. The Mayo Clinic recommends that the cardiologist perform approximately 40 endoscopic intubations under the direct supervision of a gastroenterologist or a cardiologist trained in TEE.[8] Bansal and Shah[9] recommend 25 to 40 supervised procedures to make an individual comfortable in performing these examinations independently.

In our experience, a minimum of 25 supervised TEE procedures are necessary prior to certifying a cardiologist in performing these examinations independently. To maintain competency in performing TEE,

Table 3-5. Guidelines for Training Requirements for a Cardiologist to Perform TEE

Experienced in transthoracic 2-D and Doppler techniques

Attendance of continuing medical education course or preceptorship program for TEE (see Table 3-6)

Performance of a minimum of 25 TEE procedures under direct supervision

Knowledge of indications, contraindications, and potential complications

Familiarity with biplane tomographic anatomy

the operator should continue to perform a reasonable number of cases per month. In our laboratory, we periodically review the appropriateness of the procedures and complication rates.

Anesthesiologists wishing to train in the technique must also adhere to the guidelines set up for training of cardiologists. In addition, the anesthesiologist should spend a reasonable amount of time in the echocardiography laboratory with an experienced echocardiographer to acquire competence in basic 2-D and color Doppler echocardiography.

Table 3-6. Activities to Be Incorporated in the TEE Preceptorship Program

Equipment and laboratory setup

Techniques, indications, contraindications, and potential complications

Tomographic anatomy (single plane and biplane)

Observation of TEE procedures

Informal sessions and clinical discussions

Review of teaching tapes

Intraoperative TEE, when available

TEE in the critical care unit

In the setting of a cardiology fellowship program, the trainee can obtain enough experience in all aspects of echocardiography and TEE techniques. In our institution, a fellow wishing to obtain advanced experience in echocardiography will spend most of the year training in the echocardiography laboratory and participating in clinical research. This is obviously the ideal setting for training cardiologists in this emerging technical field. However, there are many established preceptorship programs for cardiologists in practice who may wish to obtain training in TEE. Our laboratory has been instrumental in training other cardiologists in community hospitals to perform the procedure. Tables 3-5 and 3-6 list some of our guidelines for training cardiologists to perform TEE.

REFERENCES

1. Steckelberg JM, Khandheria BK, Anhalt JP, et al. Prospective evaluation of the risk of bacteremia associated with transesophageal echocardiography. Circulation 1991; 84:177–180.
2. Chandrasekaran K, Bansal RC, Ross JJ, et al. Impact of transesophageal color-flow Doppler echocardiography in current clinical cardiology practice. Echocardiography 1990; 7:125–145.
3. Dawson J, Cockel R. Oesophageal perforation at fiberoptic gastroscopy. Br Heart J 1981; 283:583.
4. Daniel WG, Erbel R, Kasper W, et al. Safety of transesophageal echocardiography. A multicenter survey of 10,419 examinations. Circulation 1991; 83:817–821.
5. Khandheria BK, Seward JB, Tajik AJ. Transesophageal Echocardiography. In Braunwald E (ed): Heart Disease Update. Philadelphia, WB Saunders, 1991.
6. O'Shea JP, Southern JF, D'Ambra MN, et al. Effects of prolonged transesophageal echocardiogtaphic imaging and probe manipulation on the esophagus—an echocardiographic-pathologic study. J Am Coll Cardiol 1991; 17:1426–1429.
7. Cucciara RF, Nugent M, Seward JB, Messick JM. Air embolism in upright neurosurgical patients: detection and localization by two-dimensional transesophageal echocardiography. Anesthesiology 1984; 60:353–355.
8. Seward JB, Khandheria BK, Oh JK, et al: Transesophageal echocardiography: technique, anatomic correlations, implementation, and clinical applications. Mayo Clin Proc 1988; 63:649–680.
9. Bansal RC, Shah PM. Transesophageal echocardiography. Curr Prob Cardiol 1990; 11:643–720.

4 Transesophageal Tomographic Anatomy

After passing the probe to the 30 to 35 cm level, it is our practice to avoid probe manipulation until the patient is fairly comfortable and not apprehensive. A comprehensive TEE examination entails a sequence of transducer positions and tomographic planes of section. Even when a specific clinical problem is being evaluated, a methodologic imaging approach comparable to that recommended for a comprehensive transthoracic echocardiographic (TTE) examination should be followed. A step-by-step approach is suggested that can be altered on the basis of the clinical situation. During TEE, two distinct tomographic examinations are performed: of the heart and of the thoracic aorta. Detailed reviews of image orientation and anatomic correlations of the tomographic sections of the heart and aorta from a transesophageal window, using a single plane and biplane probe, have been published.[1-5] Table 4-1 summarizes the various biplane TEE views. The three primary transesophageal positions using a single-plane (transverse or horizontal plane scanning) probe are illustrated in Figure 4-1; those for the longitudinal or vertical plane (using a biplane probe) are shown in Figure 4-2. During a TEE examination, sequential views of the transverse and longitudinal planes can be obtained. Simultaneous biplane images are not currently available.

CARDIAC EXAMINATION

Transverse Single-Plane Imaging

Position I: Basal Short-Axis Views

Basal short-axis planes are initially obtained, usually at 25 to 30 cm from the incisors (Figs. 4-1 and 4-3). All short-axis views display the anterior structures at the bottom of the video screen, posterior structures at the top, and left-sided structures on the viewer's right. Tilting the tips superiorly or by slightly withdrawing the transducer produces sequential basal short-axis scans. Basal short-axis scans sequentially depict the aortic valve, proximal ascending aorta, proximal coronary arteries, atrial appendages, superior vena cava, atrial septum, pulmonary veins, and proximal pulmonary arteries (Figs. 4-4 to 4-10).

The aortic valve cusps are usually imaged in the short-axis plane. The aortic root is also best seen in this view. The atrial septum with the membrane of the fossa ovalis is seen separating the left and right atria. Portions of the tricuspid valve and right ventricle may be seen in this view as well.

The origin of the left main coronary artery and its bifurcation can be seen with an upward tilt of the tip of the transducer (Fig. 4-11). The right coronary artery is somewhat difficult to image and can usually be seen at a different tomographic level, with superior or inferior tilting of the tip of the transducer (Fig. 4-12).

Superior tilting and withdrawing of the transducer 1 to 2 cm will bring into view the left atrial appendage, which appears as a triangular extension of the left atrium. Muscular ridges (pectinate muscles) within the appendage are easily visible and should not be confused with thrombi. The left atrial appendage overlies the left coronary artery. Also seen at this level is the left upper pulmonary vein, which is separated from the left atrial appendage by a distinct ridgelike infolding of the wall. The right atrial appendage is anterior to the superior vena cava.

Table 4-1. Biplane Tomographic Views

	Transverse Plane	Longitudinal Plane
Cardiac examination		
Position I: Basal views (25–30 cm)	Short-axis view of aortic valve, RVOT	Long-axis view of ascending aorta
	Coronary arteries, pulmonary veins, LAA	Long-axis view of RVOT, MPA
	Short-axis view of SVC, ascending aorta, and atrial septum	Long-axis view of SVC, atrial septum
Position II: Midesophageal views (30–35 cm)	Four-chamber view	Two-chamber view of LA, MV, LV, LAA
	Four-chamber view with LVOT	
	RV inflow and coronary sinus	
Position III: Transgastric views (35–40 cm)	Short-axis view at level of papillary muscles	Two-chamber view of LA, MV, LV
	Short-axis view of LV and MV	
Examination of the Thoracic Aorta		
	Short-axis view of thoracic aorta	Long-axis view of thoracic aorta
	Long-axis view of arch	Short-axis view of arch, brachiocephalic branches

Abbreviations: LA, left atrium; LAA, left atrial appendage; LV, left ventricle; LVOT, left ventricular outflow tract; MV, mitral valve; MPA, main pulmonary artery; RV, right ventricle; RVOT, right ventricular outflow tract; SVC, superior vena cava.

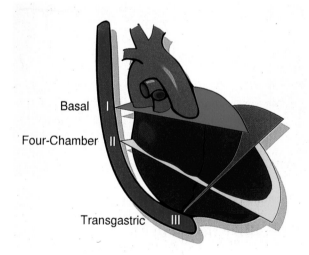

Fig. 4-1. Schematic diagram showing the commonly obtained planes obtained with the transverse or horizontal plane probe.

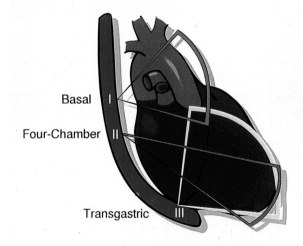

Fig. 4-2. Schematic diagram showing commonly obtained planes with the longitudinal or vertical plane probe, using a biplane TEE probe.

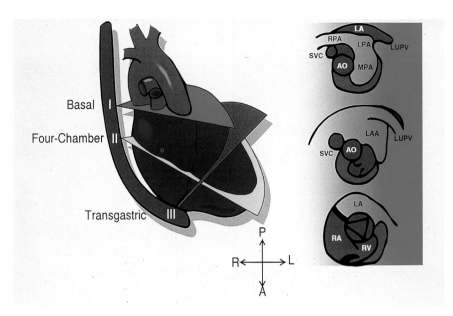

Fig. 4-3. Transverse plane from the base of the heart, position I. The diagram illustrates the various short-axis views obtained with the transducer 25 to 30 cm from the tip of the incisor teeth. A, anterior; L, left; P, posterior; R, right in the directional map; AO, aorta; LA, left atrium; LAA, left atrial appendage; LPA, left pulmonary artery; LUPV, left upper pulmonary vein; MPA, main pulmonary artery; RA, right atrium; RPA, right pulmonary artery; RV, right ventricle; SVC, superior vena cava.

Fig. 4-4. Transverse scan of aortic root. The three aortic valve cusps are evident (L, left; N, non-; R, right coronary cusps). LA, left atrium; RV, right ventricle.

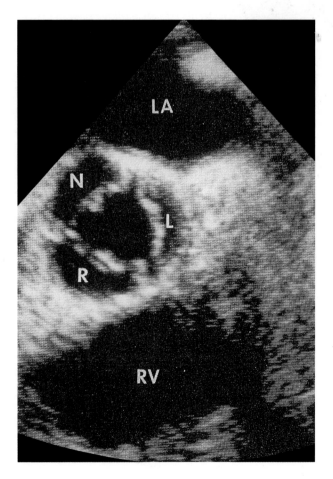

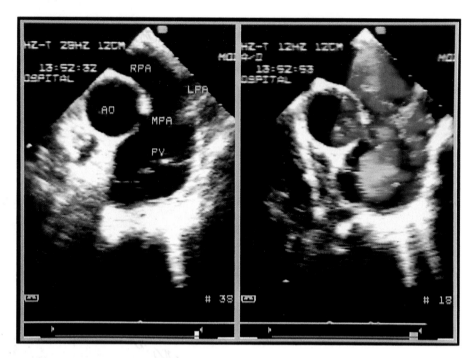

Fig. 4-5. *(Left)* Transverse basal short-axis scan of main pulmonary artery (MPA) and bifurcation. *(Right)* Color Doppler image. AO, aorta; LPA, left pulmonary artery; PV, pulmonary valve; RPA, right pulmonary artery.

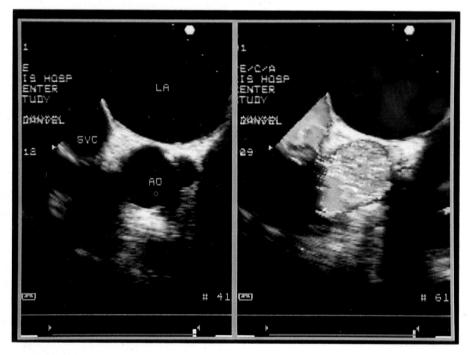

Fig. 4-6. *(Left)* Transverse basal short-axis scan of superior vena cava (SVC) and aortic root (AO). *(Right)* Color Doppler image. LA, left atrium.

Fig. 4-7. Transverse basal short-axis scan of left atrial appendage (LAA). AO, aorta; LA, left atrium.

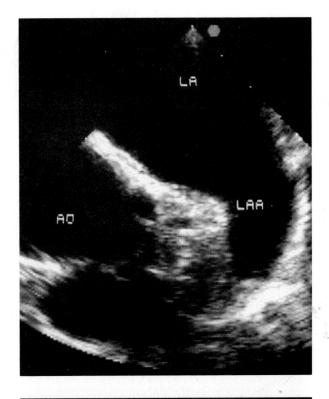

Fig. 4-8. Transverse basal short-axis scan of left atrial appendage (LAA). The pectinate muscles are frequently visible as small ridges within the appendage. AO, aorta; LA, left atrium.

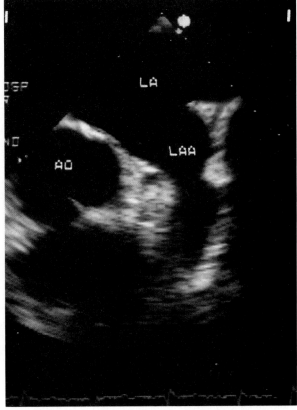

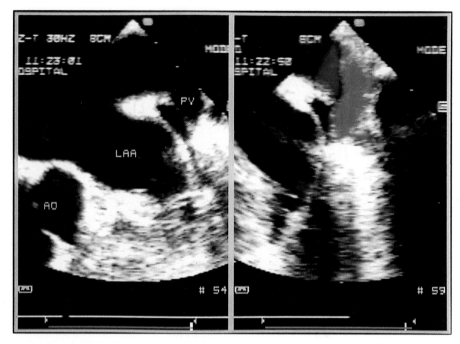

Fig. 4-9. *(Left)* Transverse basal short-axis scan of left atrial appendage (LAA) and left upper pulmonary vein (PV). The structures are separated by a ridgelike infolding of the wall. *(Right)* Pulmonary vein flow is seen as red in the color Doppler image.

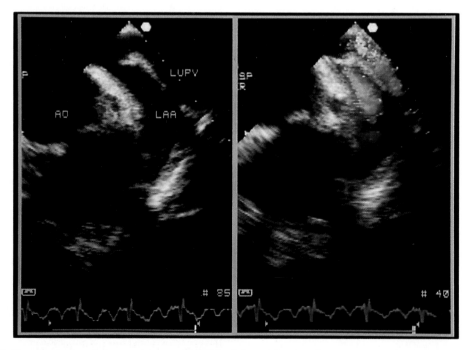

Fig. 4-10. Transverse basal short-axis scan. *(Left)* The left atrial appendage (LAA) and left upper pulmonary vein (LUPV) are separated by a ridgelike structure. *(Right)* Color Doppler image showing forward flow in the LUPV and reverse flow in the LAA. AO, aorta.

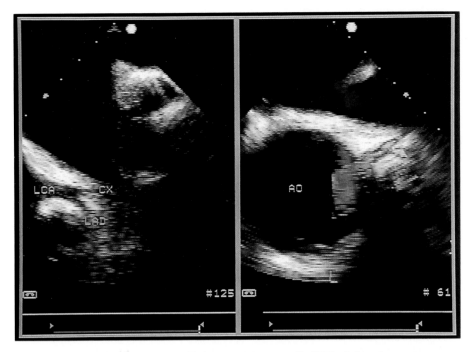

Fig. 4-11. Transverse basal short-axis scan of left coronary artery. *(Left)* The left main coronary artery (LCA) is imaged just above the left aortic cusp. Bifurcation into circumflex artery (CX) (posterior) and left anterior descending coronary artery (LAD) (anterior) is shown. *(Right)* Color Doppler image in diastole showing flow in the LCA, CX, and LAD.

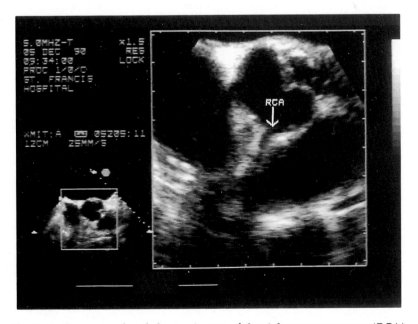

Fig. 4-12. Transverse basal short-axis scan of the right coronary artery (RCA).

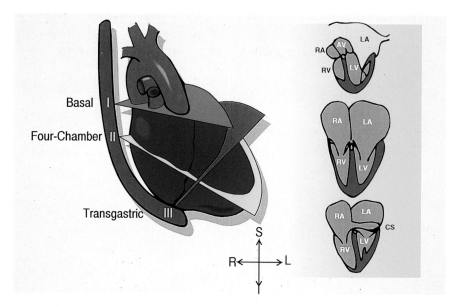

Fig. 4-13. Transverse plane from the midesophageal, position II. The views obtained include the four-chamber, four-chamber with left ventricular outflow tract and aorta (five-chamber), and coronary sinus (CS) views. I, inferior; L, left; R, right; S, superior in the directional map; AV, aortic valve; LA, left atrium; LV, left ventricle; RA, right atrium; RV, right ventricle.

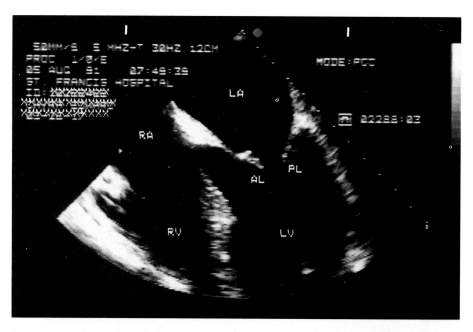

Fig. 4-14. Transverse midesophageal or four-chamber view. All four cardiac chambers are imaged simultaneously along with respective septa and atrioventricular valve. AL, anterior mitral leaflet; LA, left atrium; LV, left ventricle; PL, posterior mitral leaflet; RA, right atrium; RV, right ventricle.

The superior vena cava appears as an ovoid structure adjacent to the ascending aorta. The right upper pulmonary vein courses posteriorly and is orthogonal to the superior vena cava.

The atrial septum can be imaged from multiple short-axis and four-chamber transesophageal tomographic projections. The thin membrane of the fossa ovalis may also be imaged on the left atrial surface of the atrial septal limbus. In most patients, a complete scan of the atrial septum can be obtained from the transverse and longitudinal tomographic projections.

Position II: Midesophageal Four-Chamber Views

With further advancement of the endoscope into the esophagus to approximately 30 to 35 cm from the incisors and the tip slightly retroflexed, four-chamber plane tomographic views of the heart are obtained (Figs. 4-13 and 4-14). These tomographic scans image the atrioventricular valves and support apparatus, ventricles, left ventricular outflow tract, and coronary sinus. Color Doppler assessment for regurgitation of atrioventricular and aortic valves is performed from this transducer position. As per the recommendations of the American Society of Echocardiography,[3] the four-chamber view is displayed with the apex down, with the left ventricle on the viewer's right and the right ventricle on the viewer's left.

From the four-chamber recording position, progressive anteflexion will display the left ventricular outflow tract and the long axis of the aortic valve and aorta, similar to the transthoracic apical five-chamber view (Fig. 4-15). Slight advancement and extreme retroflexion of the tip from the four-chamber recording position will display the right ventricular inflow and long axis of the coronary sinus (Fig. 4-16).

Anatomic and functional abnormalities of the mitral annulus, leaflets, and subvalvular apparatus can be readily imaged in this four-chamber plane of section.

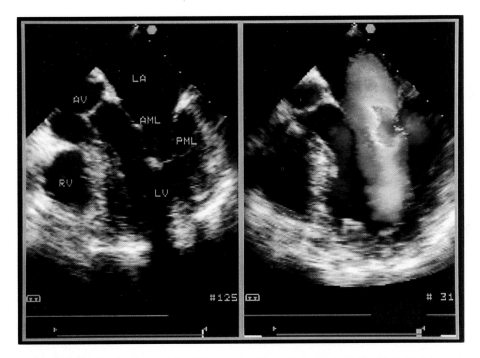

Fig. 4-15. Transverse long-axis view of the left ventricular outflow tract. *(Left)* Diastolic frame showing the anterior mitral leaflet (AML) and posterior mitral leaflet (PML) and the long-axis of the left ventricular outflow tract and aortic valve (AV). *(Right)* Color Doppler image of left ventricular inflow. LA, left atrium; LV, left ventricle; RV, portion of right ventricular inflow.

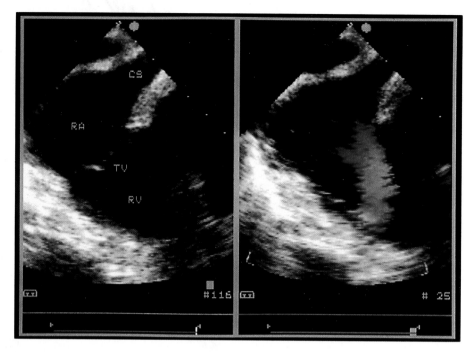

Fig. 4-16. Transverse long-axis view of coronary sinus (CS). *(Left)* The right atrium (RA), right ventricle (RV) and tricuspid valve (TV) are visible when scan is optimized for coronary sinus. *(Right)* Color Doppler image depicting right ventricular inflow.

Although the anterolateral papillary muscle is most frequently imaged in the anterior four-chamber plane, the posteromedial papillary muscle can be visualized only with extreme retroflexion of the endoscope. Because the mitral valve orifice is parallel to the ultrasound beam in this view, excellent pulsed and continuous-wave Doppler and color Doppler imaging examinations can be performed.

Tricuspid valve leaflets are also imaged in the long-axis projection; however, the orifice is oblique to the plane of section. Because the orifice is off axis, an accurate Doppler examination cannot be performed without angle correction. The longitudinal plane appears to be more reliable in obtaining an accurate pulsed and continuous-wave Doppler examination without angle correction. Color Doppler imaging, however, can be used to evaluate tricuspid valve regurgitation semiquantitatively. Tomographic sections from the four-chamber planes also permit assessment of the atria, atrial septum, and internal crux of the heart (Figs. 4-17 and 4-18).

Position III: Transgastric Short-Axis Views

With the endoscope controls in a neutral and unlocked position, the instrument is advanced at approximately 35 to 40 cm from the incisors into the stomach and anteflexed to image the short axis of the heart from the fundus of the stomach and the left lobe of the liver (Fig. 4-19). At this level, images of the papillary muscles and mitral valve orifice are obtained (Fig. 4-20). These views are used to assess left ventricular function and, intraoperatively, to monitor global and regional myocardial function.

We display the left ventricle to the right and the right ventricle to the left, an orientation similar to that recommended by the American Society of Echocardiog-

Fig. 4-17. Transverse four-chamber view of atrial septum. The thin valve of fossa ovalis (arrows) can be consistently imaged. LA, left atrium; RA, right atrium.

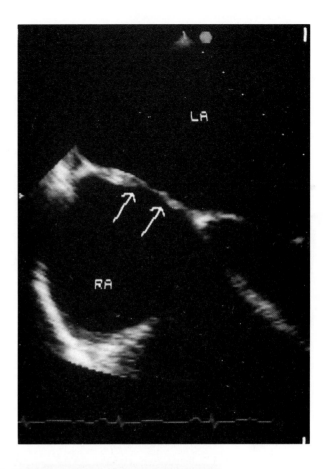

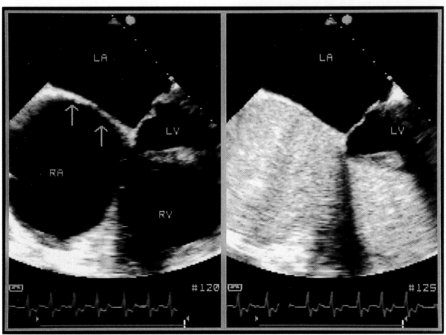

Fig. 4-18. *(Left)* Transverse four-chamber view of atrial septum (arrows). *(Right)* Normal contrast study (agitated saline) opacifies the right atrium (RA) and right ventricle (RV) and delineates the right side of the atrial septum. No evidence of contrast in the left atrium (LA). LV, left ventricle.

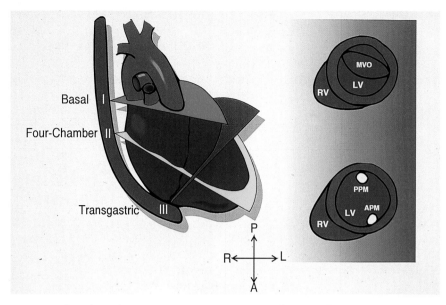

Fig. 4-19. Transverse plane from the transgastric, position III. The diagram illustrates the transgastric short-axis views at the level of the mitral valve and at the level of the papillary muscles. A, anterior; L, left; P, posterior; R, right in the directional map; APM, anterior papillary muscle; LV, left ventricle; MVO, mitral valve orifice; PPM, posteromedical papillary muscle; RV, right ventricle.

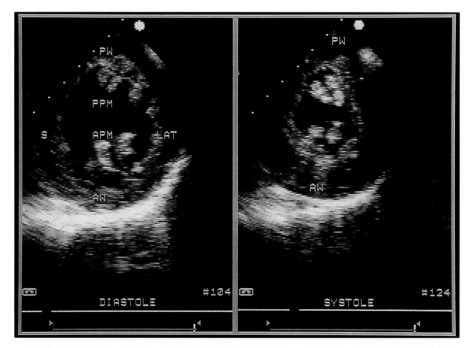

Fig. 4-20. Transgastric short-axis view at the level of the papillary muscles; systolic and diastolic frames. APM, anterior papillary muscle; AW, anterior wall of left ventricle; LAT, lateral wall of left ventricle; PPM, posteromedial papillary muscle; PW, posterior wall of left ventricle; S, ventricular septum.

raphy for display of ventricular short-axis views. Posterior structures are viewed at the top of the screen and the anterior structures at the bottom.

Biplane Longitudinal Imaging (Fig. 4-2)

Position I: Basal Views

After completion of the basal short-axis views using the transverse plane probe (Fig. 4-21), changing to the long-axis plane probe with slight clockwise rotation of the shaft will provide a long-axis view of the ascending aorta (Fig. 4-22). Counterclockwise rotation of the probe will also provide visualization of the right ventricular outflow tract, pulmonic valve, and main pulmonary artery from the long-axis scanning probe (Fig. 4-23). The transverse plane probe displays the superior vena cava and ascending aorta in the short axis. Changing to the longitudinal plane probe at this level will permit visualization of the superior vena cava in the long axis and of the entire

atrial septum (Fig. 4-24). Advancement of the scope permits imaging of the eustachian valve and proximal inferior vena cava in the long axis (Fig. 4-25).

The tomographic views obtained by the long-axis scanning transducer display the posterior structures either at the top of the video screen or on the viewer's left, the anterior structures either at the bottom of the video screen or on the viewer's right, and the superior structures either on the viewer's right or at the top of the screen. Some institutions alter the longitudinal plane images electronically to simulate the images obtained by TTE.

Longitudinal imaging is superior to transverse imaging for visualization of the aortic cusps and the proximal and distal portions of the ascending aorta. The "blind" area,[2] representing the upper portion of the ascending aorta in the transverse plane (caused by the interposed air-filled trachea and bronchi), is almost eliminated in the longitudinal scanning plane.

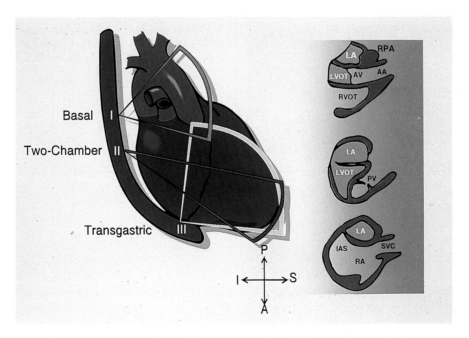

Fig. 4-21. Longitudinal plane from the base of the heart, position I. The diagram depicts the various long-axis views from the base of the heart. A, anterior; I, inferior; P, posterior; S, superior in the directional map. AA, ascending aorta; AV, aortic valve; IAS, interatrial septum; LA, left atrium; LVOT, left ventricular outflow tract; PV, pulmonary valve; RA, right atrium; RPA, right pulmonary artery; RVOT, right ventricular outflow tract; SVC, superior vena cava.

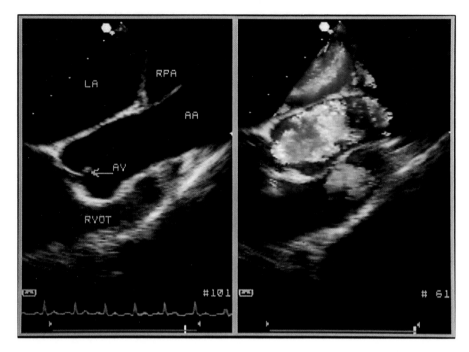

Fig. 4-22. Longitudinal basal view. *(Left)* The ascending aorta (AA) is visualized in long-axis view. Posterior to AA is the right pulmonary artery (RPA). *(Right)* Color Doppler image in systole demonstrating flow in the AA. AV, aortic valve; LA, left atrium; RVOT, right ventricular outflow tract.

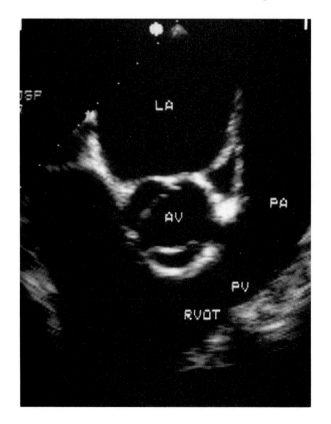

Fig. 4-23. Longitudinal basal view of right ventricular outflow tract (RVOT), pulmonary valve (PV), and main pulmonary artery (PA). AV, aortic valve; LA, left atrium.

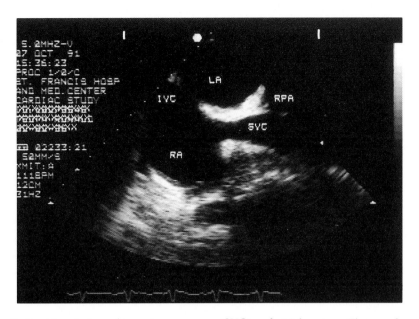

Fig. 4-24. Longitudinal basal view of superior vena cava (SVC) and atrial septum. The membrane of the fossa ovalis is seen as a thin membranous structure. IVC, inferior vena cava; LA, left atrium; RA, right atrium; RPA, right pulmonary artery.

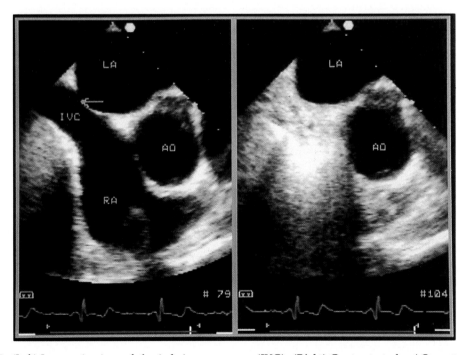

Fig. 4-25. *(Left)* Long-axis view of the inferior vena cava (IVC). *(Right)* Contrast study. AO, aorta; LA, left atrium; RA, right atrium.

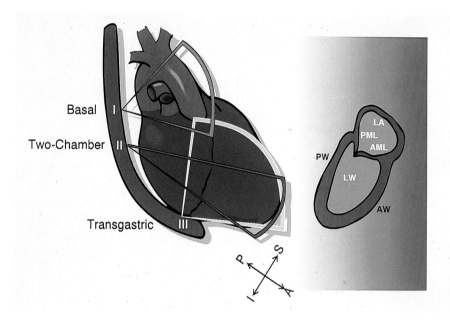

Fig. 4-26. Longitudinal plane at the midesophageal, position II. The diagram illustrates the two-chamber view. A, anterior; I, inferior; P, posterior; S, superior in the directional map; AML, lateral segment of anterior mitral leaflet; AW, anterior wall of left ventricle; LA, left atrium; LV, left ventricle; PML, middle scallop of posterior mitral leaflet; PW, posterior wall of left ventricle.

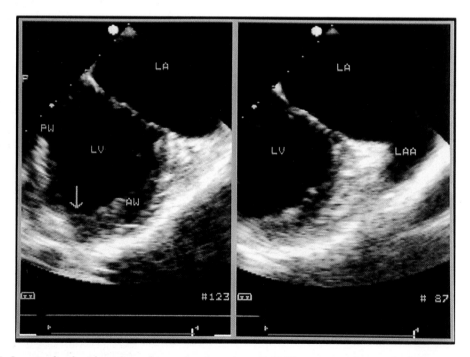

Fig. 4-27. Longitudinal midesophageal two-chamber view. *(Left)* The arrow points to the left ventricular (LV) apex. *(Right)* Slight clockwise rotation of the probe reveals the left atrial appendage (LAA). AW, anterior wall; LA, left atrium; PW, posterior wall.

The right ventricular outflow tract, pulmonary valve, and main pulmonary artery are also optimally visualized in the longitudinal scanning plane. Visualization of the distal portion of both right and left pulmonary arteries is enhanced with longitudinal imaging.

Biplanar imaging is far superior to single plane imaging for delineation of atrial septal anatomy. Views of the atrial septum in particular, the valve of the fossa ovalis and the superior and inferior limbi of the atrial septum, are optimally obtained with the longitudinal scanning plane.

Position II: Midesophageal Two-Chamber View

From position II, the transverse scanning plane probe permits sectioning through the four-chamber plane, and the longitudinal scan probe permits assessment of the left atrium and left ventricle in the two-chamber view from the midesophageal position (Figs. 4-26 and 4-27). This section transects the left atrium, mitral valve orifice, and portions of the left ventricular inflow tract. The left atrial appendage and left upper pulmonary vein are visualized to the right of the video screen.

In order to image the left ventricular outflow tract in the long axis, the tip of the scope is flexed leftward, with medial rotation of the tip of the scope, to optimize this long-axis view of the left ventricular outflow tract, aortic valve, and aortic root (Fig. 4-28).

Position III: Transgastric Two-Chamber View

From the transgastric position III, the transverse plane transducer permits viewing of the left ventricle

Fig. 4-28. Long-axis view of the left ventricular outflow tract (LVOT). The right ventricular outflow tract (RVOT) and main pulmonary artery (PA) are also visualized. LA, left atrium.

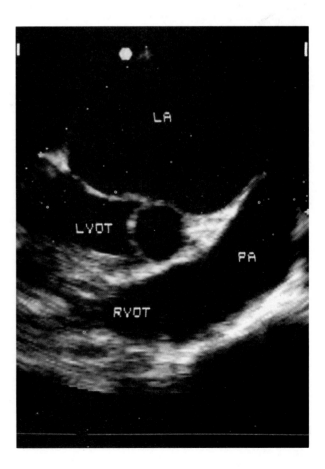

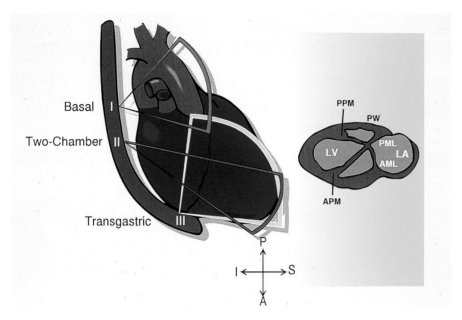

Fig. 4-29. Longitudinal plane from the transgastric, position III. The diagram shows the transgastric two-chamber view. A, anterior; I, inferior; P, posterior; S, superior in the directional map; AML, lateral segment of anterior mitral leaflet; APM, anterior papillary muscle; AW, anterior wall of left ventricle; LA, left atrium; LV, left ventricle; PML, medial scallop of posterior mitral leaflet; PPM, posteromedial papillary muscle; PW, posterior wall of left ventricle.

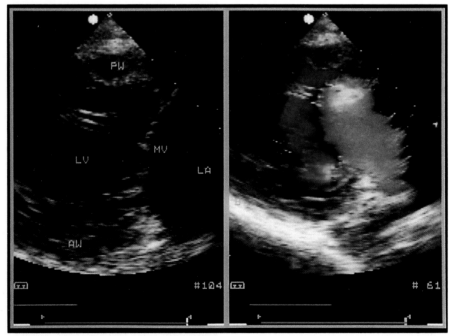

Fig. 4-30. Longitudinal transgastric scan of the left heart. *(Left)* Two-chamber view of the left atrium (LA) and left ventricle (LV). *(Right)* Color Doppler image of LV inflow. AW, anterior wall; MV, mitral valve; PW, posterior wall.

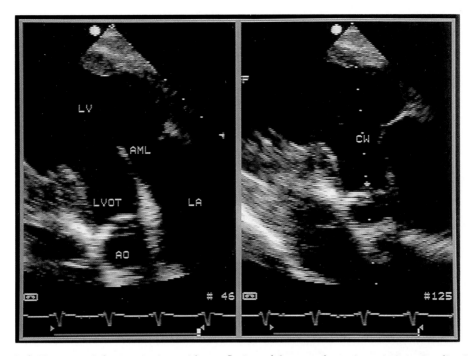

Fig. 4-31. *(Left)* Transgastric long-axis view with anteflexion of the transducer tip optimizes visualization of the left ventricular outflow tract (LVOT) and aortic valve. *(Right)* This view permits parallel alignment of continuous-wave (CW) Doppler beam in the LVOT for assessment of obstructions at subvalvular and valvular levels. AO, aorta; AML, anterior mitral valve leaflet; LA, left atrium; LV, left ventricle.

in the short axis (Fig. 4-29) and the longitudinal plane transducer permits a long-axis or transgastric two-chamber view (Fig. 4-30). The left ventricular apex is often best appreciated by transgastric longitudinal plane imaging. For optimal long-axis orientation, slight leftward or rightward flexion and rotation of the tip of the endoscope may be necessary. Anteflexion of the tip produces an apical long-axis equivalent view of the left ventricle and aortic and mitral valves (Fig. 4-31). This view should be ideal for transesophageal continuous-wave Doppler assessment of aortic stenosis and regurgitation.

Limitations of Biplane Imaging

Minor limitations of the biplane probe include (1) the need for minimal repositioning of the tip when changing from the transverse to the longitudinal plane probe because the two transducers are separated by 1 cm, and (2) a display of both images simultaneously from cine-loop memory in a non-real-time format. Current research designed to overcome these problems includes the development of a matrix phased-array probe.[6]

EXAMINATION OF THE THORACIC AORTA

The upper ascending aorta, aortic arch, proximal brachiocephalic vessel, and descending aorta can be comprehensively imaged in both the transverse and the longitudinal planes (Fig. 4-32). Biplanar imaging complements the overall assessment of aortic pathologic conditions.

Visualization of the ascending aorta using the transverse and longitudinal plane imaging has been previously described. The shaft of the echoscope is rotated slightly counterclockwise (behind the left atrium) to visualize the cross section of the midthoracic descending aorta, using the transverse plane

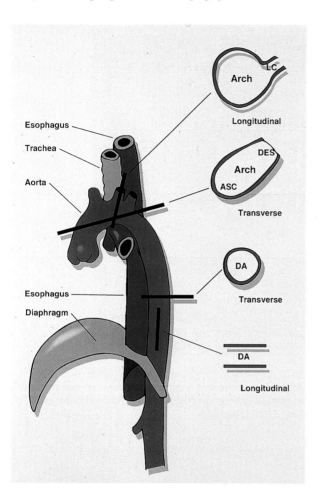

Fig. 4-32. Schematic diagram of the relationship of the aorta to the esophagus as they course from the thorax to the abdomen. The various planes and views of the aortic arch and descending thoracic aorta (DA) are shown on the right, using the transverse and longitudinal plane views. ASC, ascending portion of arch; DES, descending portion of arch; LC, left carotid artery.

scanning transducer. The echoscope is then gradually advanced into the stomach (approximately 50 cm from incisors), while keeping the aorta in view. Slight anteflexion of the tip of the echoscope provides better contact of the transducer with the esophagus. The probe is gradually withdrawn in 5-cm increments, while keeping the aorta in view to examine the upper abdominal and entire descending thoracic aorta in both the transverse and longitudinal planes (Fig. 4-33). The mid- and distal abdominal aorta cannot be seen because of difficulty in maintaining good contact between the esophageal transducer and the mucosa of the stomach. The examiner must record the depth in centimeters from the incisors at the regions of aortic pathology.

The arch can be imaged by slowly withdrawing the probe to about 18 to 20 cm (Fig. 4-34). As the tip of the echoscope approaches the posterior pharynx, the gag and cough reflexes will increase, causing the patient discomfort and preventing prolonged imaging in this position. Since the aortic arch lies slightly anterior to the esophagus, the operator, while withdrawing the scope from the midthoracic aorta, should rotate the probe slightly clockwise, or to the patient's right. With the transverse plane scanning probe, the arch is displayed in its long-axis view with the ascending arch on the left of the screen. The left common carotid artery and the proximal portion of the left subclavian artery may also be seen as the echoscope is withdrawn superior to the aortic arch. The

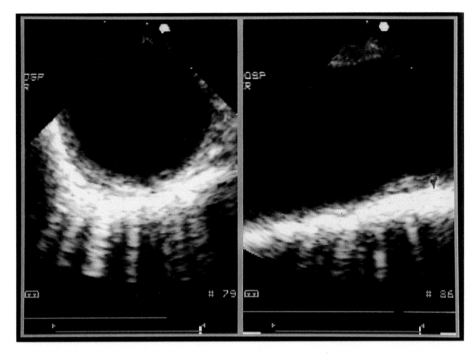

Fig. 4-33. *(Left)* Transverse plane of the descending thoracic aorta. *(Right)* Longitudinal plane of the descending aorta obtained from the same probe position.

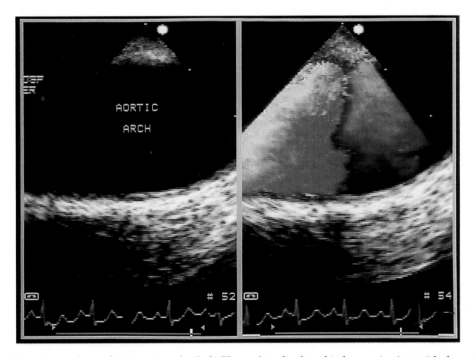

Fig. 4-34. Transverse plane of the aortic arch. *(Left)* The arch is displayed in long-axis view with the ascending portion of the arch on the left. *(Right)* Color Doppler image showing the ascending portion of the arch in red and the descending portion of the arch in blue.

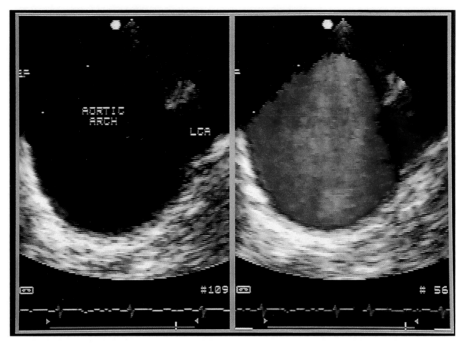

Fig. 4-35. *(Left)* Longitudinal scan of the aortic arch with visualization of the left common carotid artery (LCA). *(Right)* Color Doppler imaging of the aortic arch (red) and LCA (dark blue).

right innominate artery cannot be seen because of the air-filled trachea. When the echoscope is superior to the arch, the tip should be rotated counterclockwise to scan the long axis of the left subclavian artery, coursing away from the transducer on the left lower portion of the video screen. The left common carotid may be seen in its short axis on the medial side of the left subclavian artery and the left jugular vein anterior to the left common carotid artery at the bottom the video screen.

From the aortic arch position, switching to the longitudinal plane scanning transducer, the short axis of the arch with one of the brachiocephalic vessels in its long axis (commonly the left carotid) is often recorded (Fig. 4-35). Rotation of the shaft of the transducer often permits visualization of all three vessels, especially in cases with dilated arches.

REFERENCES

1. Schlüter M, Hinrichs A, Their W, et al. Transesophageal two-dimensional echocardiography: comparison of ultrasonic and anatomic sections. Am J Cardiol 1984; 53:1173–1178.
2. Seward JB, Khandheria BK, Oh JK, et al. Transesophageal echocardiography: technique, anatomic correlations, implementation and clinical applications. Mayo Clin Proc 1988; 63:649–680.
3. Schiller NB, Maurer G, Ritter SB, et al. Transesophageal echocardiography. J Am Soc Echocardiol 1989; 2:354–357.
4. Seward JB, Khandheria BK, Edwards WD, et al. Biplanar transesophageal echocardiography: anatomic correlations, image orientation, and clinical applications. Mayo Clin Proc 1990; 65:1193–1213.
5. Richardson SG, Weintraub AR, Schwartz SL, et al. Biplane Transesophageal echocardiography utilizing transverse and sagittal imaging planes: technique, echo-anatomic correlations, and display approaches. Echocardiography 1991; 8:293–309.
6. Omoto R, Kyo S, Matsumura M, et al. Biplane color Doppler transesophageal echocardiography: its impact on cardiovascular surgery and further technological progress in the probe, a matrix phased-array biplane probe. Echocardiography 1989; 6:423–430.

5 Assessment of Aortic Valve Disease

Evaluation of aortic regurgitation and stenosis of native or prosthetic aortic valve are generally well visualized from the parasternal imaging planes by transthoracic echocardiography (TTE) in most patients. Because the aortic valve is imaged at an oblique angle with single-plane TEE using the transverse views, accurate Doppler and color Doppler information add little to the transthoracic examination. However, because of the relatively superior image quality, TEE often adds valuable information to the precordial examination by providing more frequent delineation of the underlying pathology of aortic regurgitation. In addition, a significant proportion of patients offer technically inadequate parasternal imaging attributable to musculoskeletal or pulmonary pathologies.

The advent of biplane imaging has permitted a more accurate assessment of the aortic root and valve in most patients. Biplane imaging of the aortic valve and of the root permits assessment of the number of aortic cusps (unicuspid, bicuspid, tricuspid, or quadricuspid), of the size of the aortic root, dissection, and of aortic valve endocarditis and its complications. Aortic aneurysms and dissections, valvular endocarditis, and prosthetic valve dysfunction are discussed in subsequent chapters.

AORTIC REGURGITATION

The normal aortic valve is well visualized in the transverse and longitudinal planes. The valve is formed by three nearly equal cusps (see Ch. 4, Fig. 4-4). The left cusp is displayed on the viewer's right, the right cusp to the left and inferiorly and the noncoronary cusp to the left and above the right coronary cusp. The three-valve cusps are thin and should coapt during diastole while opening well to the periphery of the aorta during systole.

In the transverse plane, aortic regurgitation is detected using the basal views at the level of the aortic valve (Figs. 5-1 to 5-3) and at the midesophageal position in the five-chamber view (left ventricular outflow tract view) (Figs. 5-4 to 5-6). Using the longitudinal plane, aortic regurgitation is seen when the transducer is imaging the long axis of the aorta and left ventricular outflow tract (Figs. 5-7 and 5-8). Aortic regurgitant flow striking the anterior mitral valve leaflet may produce a characteristic flutter that is easily seen on M-mode recordings. The aortic regurgitant jet can arise from the central point of the valve, where the leaflets coapt; at other times, an eccentric jet passing through a torn or prolapsed cusp may be seen. The basal short-axis image may help determine which cusp is torn and which cusp is prolapsing.

Despite the increase in application of TEE, few data exist on the presence and size of flow disturbances visualized from this approach compared with the transthoracic window. Smith and co-workers[1] have compared aortic regurgitant jet areas by color Doppler imaging derived from the transesophageal approach with measurements obtained from conventional transthoracic apical views. Their data demonstrate that aortic regurgitant jet areas depicted by

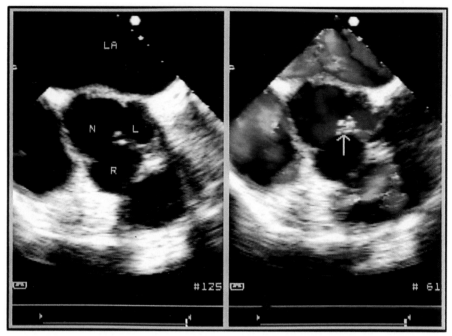

Fig. 5-1. *(Left)* Transverse basal short-axis view showing three aortic valve cusps (L, left; N, non-; R, right) in patient with hypertension. *(Right)* Color Doppler image of mild aortic regurgitation (arrow). LA, left atrium.

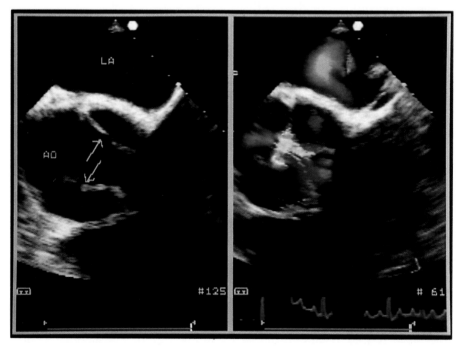

Fig. 5-2. Transverse basal short-axis view. *(Left)* Bicuspid aortic valve (arrows). *(Right)* Color Doppler image revealing mild aortic regurgitation. AO, aorta; LA, left atrium.

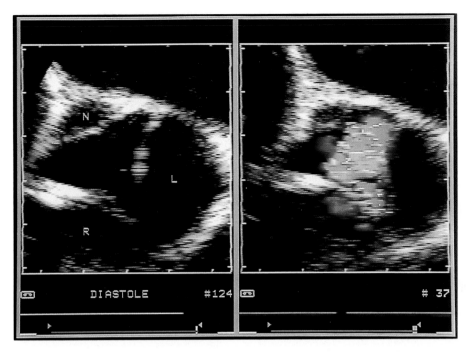

Fig. 5-3. Transverse basal short-axis view. *(Left)* Diastolic frame demonstrating incomplete coaptation of valve cusps in patient with dilated aortic root. *(Right)* Color Doppler image of moderate to severe aortic regurgitation. L, left cusp; N, noncoronary cusp; R, right cusp.

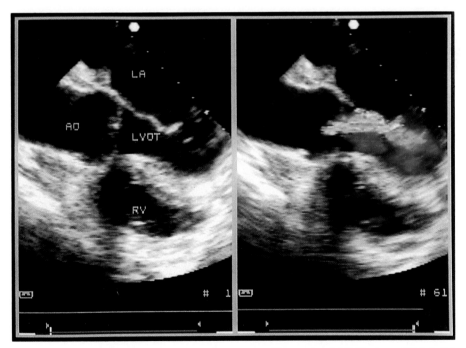

Fig. 5-4. *(Left)* Transverse midesophageal left ventricular outflow tract (LVOT) view. *(Right)* Color Doppler image demonsrating aortic regurgitation striking the anterior mitral valve leaflet. AO, aorta; LA, left atrium; RV, right ventricle.

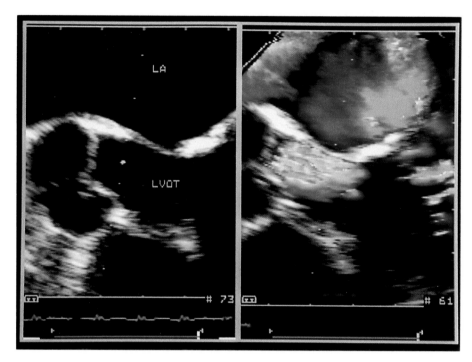

Fig. 5-5. *(Left)* Transverse left ventricular outflow tract (LVOT) view. *(Right)* Color Doppler image of moderate aortic regurgitation. LA, left atrium.

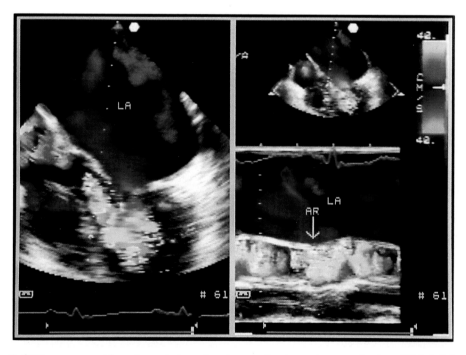

Fig. 5-6. *(Left)* Transverse midesophageal view showing moderate aortic regurgitation. *(Right)* Color M-mode demonstrating aortic regurgitation (AR). LA, left atrium.

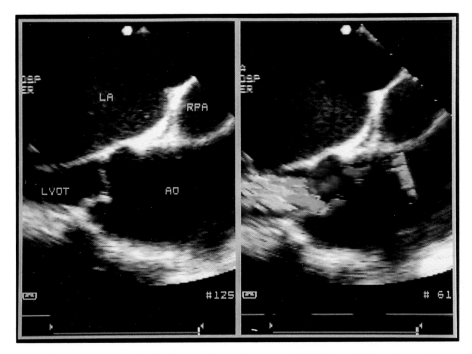

Fig. 5-7. *(Left)* Longitudinal plane of left ventricular outflow tract (LVOT), and dilated ascending aorta (AO). *(Right)* Color Doppler image of severe aortic regurgitation. LA, left atrium; RPA, right pulmonary artery.

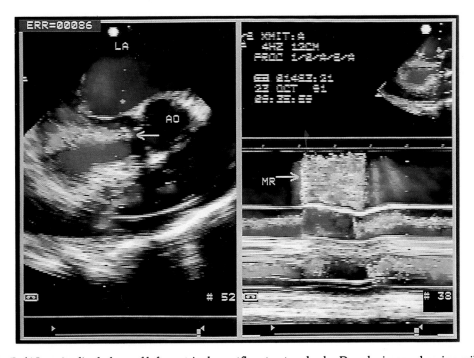

Fig. 5-8. *(Left)* Longitudinal plane of left ventricular outflow tract and color Doppler image showing mild aortic regurgitation (arrow). Mild pulmonary valve regurgitation (blue) is seen along with pulmonary artery catheter (linear density). *(Right)* Color M-mode demonstrating aortic regurgitation, pulmonic regurgitation and mitral regurgitation (MR). AO, aorta; LA, left atrium.

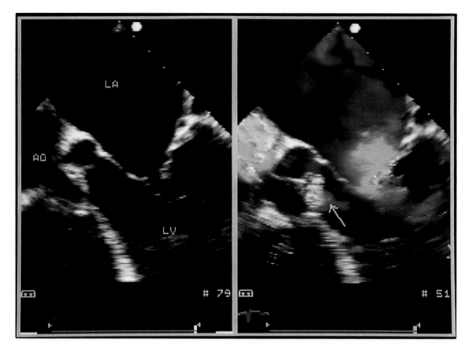

Fig. 5-9. Mild aortic regurgitation. *(Left)* Transverse midesophageal view of left ventricular outflow tract. *(Right)* Color Doppler mapping shows aortic regurgitation (arrow). AO, aorta; LA, left atrium; LV, left ventricle.

transesophageal color Doppler imaging are larger than those portrayed by transthoracic imaging. As this study failed to determine the true sensitivity and specificity for transesophageal and transthoracic flow mapping in identifying and quantifying aortic regurgitation, currently used standards for predicting severity of aortic regurgitation by color Doppler mapping must be reexamined when the esophageal window is used.

Unpublished data from our laboratory have shown a good correlation between aortic regurgitation severity by TEE color Doppler imaging and that determined angiographically from the ratio of the regurgitant jet diameter at its origin to left ventricular outflow tract diameter (Figs. 5-9 to 5-13). These findings are similar to that of Perry et al.,[2] who reported similar findings using transthoracic color Doppler mapping.

It should be noted that mapping the jet width in relationship to the width of the left ventricular outflow tract to estimate the severity of aortic regurgitation is influenced by image quality, gain settings, and flow masking by prosthetic valves or calcification within the native valve or annulus, which may limit visualization of the entire regurgitant jet. The use of the biplane transesophageal transducer may eliminate these imaging difficulties by offering additional scan planes for jet visualization in orthogonal views.

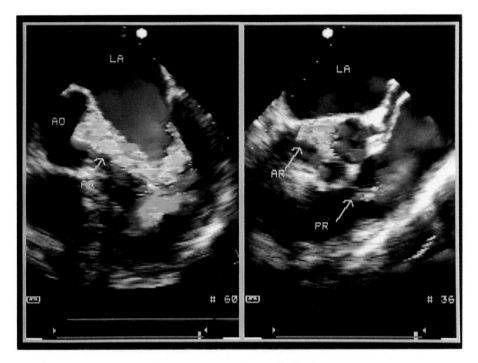

Fig. 5-10. Biplane imaging of moderate aortic regurgitation (AR). *(Left)* Transverse plane. *(Right)* Longitudinal plane. There is also pulmonary valve regurgitation (PR). AO, aorta; LA, left atrium.

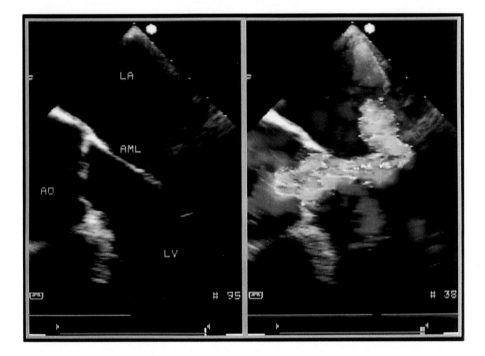

Fig. 5-11. Moderate aortic regurgitation. *(Left)* Transverse view of left ventricular outflow tract. *(Right)* Aortic regurgitant jet striking the anterior mitral valve leaflet (AML). AO, aorta; LA, left atrium; LV, left ventricle.

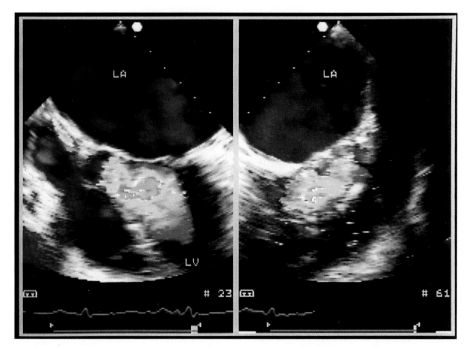

Fig. 5-12. Biplane imaging of severe aortic regurgitation. *(Left)* Transverse plane. *(Right)* Longitudinal plane. LA, left atrium; LV, left ventricle.

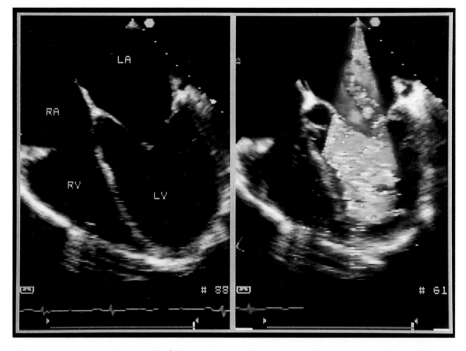

Fig. 5-13. Severe aortic regurgitation. *(Left)* Transverse midesophageal five-chamber view. The left atrium (LA) and left ventricle (LV) are enlarged. *(Right)* Color Doppler image of severe aortic regurgitation filling the entire left ventricular cavity. RA, right atrium; RV, right ventricle.

AORTIC STENOSIS

In most patients with aortic stenosis, conventional transthoracic echo-Doppler examination using continuous-wave Doppler information to derive the peak, instantaneous, and mean gradients and aortic valve area by the continuity equation for stenosis severity usually yields adequate results for clinical decision making. In approximately 10 percent to 15 percent of patients, TTE cannot quantify aortic valve gradients reliably, primarily for anatomic reasons. In these patients, however, TEE has been reported to be reliable in the determination of aortic valve area.[3] The transgastric apical long-axis view of the left ventricle and aortic and mitral valves (see Ch. 4, Fig. 4-31) should be ideal for transesophageal continuous-wave Doppler assessment of aortic stenosis.

Determination of aortic valve area is performed by planimetry using the basal short-axis view of the aortic valve in early systole.[3] The valve orifice cannot be measured in all cases, however, especially when valves are severely calcified and no orifice area can be found. However, even in those cases in which the orifice cannot be measured, the transesophageal approach permits evaluation of the morphology of the valves and their mobility during the cardiac cycle, as well as differentiation between sclerosis and stenosis (Figs. 5-14 and 5-15).

TEE is useful for distinguishing among fibromuscular ring, left ventricular outflow tract tunnel, and localized left ventricular outflow tract septal hypertrophy, and for location of the primary left ventricular outflow tract pressure gradient in hypertrophic obstructive cardiomyopathy.[4-6] It is also an excellent tech-

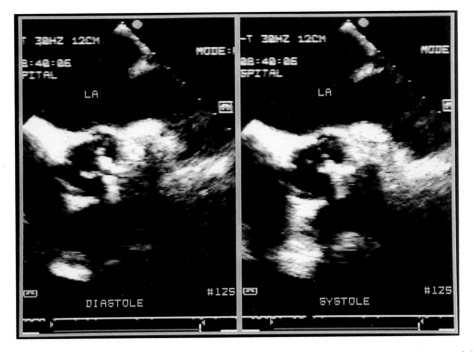

Fig. 5-14. Transverse basal short-axis view of severe aortic stenosis. Note the extensive calcification of the aortic valve and restricted mobility. LA, left atrium.

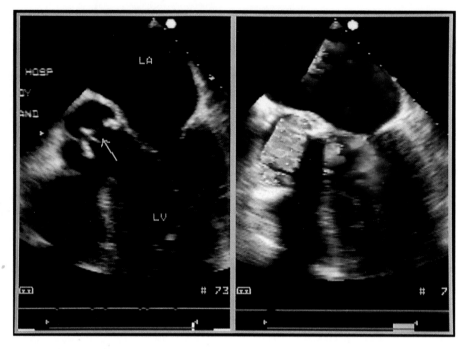

Fig. 5-15. Aortic stenosis. *(Left)* Transverse midesophageal view demonstrating calcified aortic valve (arrow) and restricted mobility. *(Right)* Color Doppler image shows turbulent flow in the aorta characteristic of aortic stenosis. LA, left atrium; LV, left ventricle.

nique for the diagnosis of subaortic obstruction and supraaortic stenosis in hypercalcemia.[7] In addition, TEE has been used during balloon aortic valvuloplasty to assess for residual aortic regurgitation, integrity of the aortic root, and degree of disruption of the aortic valve leaflets.[8]

REFERENCES

1. Smith MD, Harrison MR, Pinton R, et al. Regurgitant jet size by transesophageal compared with transthoracic Doppler color flow imaging. Circulation 1991; 83:79–86.
2. Perry GJ, Helmcke F, Nanda NC, et al. Evaluation of aortic insufficiency by Doppler color flow mapping. J Am Coll Cardiol 1987; 9:952–959.
3. Hofmann T, Kasper W, Meinertz T, et al. Determination of aortic valve orifice area in aortic valve stenosis by two-dimensional transesophageal echocardiography. Am J Cardiol 1987; 59:330–335.
4. Roelandt J. Colour-coded Doppler flow imaging: What are the prospects? Eur Heart J 1986; 7:184–189.
5. Bommer WJ, Miller L. Real-time two-dimensional color-flow Doppler. Enhanced Doppler flow imaging in the diagnosis of cardiovascular disease. Am J Cardiol 1982; 49:944 (abstract).
6. Miyataka K, Okamoto M, Kinoshita N, et al. Clinical applications of a new type of real-time two-dimensional flow imaging system. Am J Cardiol 1984; 54:857–868.
7. Cahalan M, Litt L, Botinick E, et al. Advances in noninvasive cardiovascular imaging: implications for the anesthesiologist. Anesthesiology 1987; 66:356–368.
8. Cyran SE, Kimball TR, Schwartz DC, et al. Am Heart J 1988; 115:460–462.

6 Evaluation of Mitral Regurgitation and Other Mitral Diseases

Although conventional transthoracic echocardiography (TTE) usually provides adequate information on the structure and function of the mitral valve, TEE, by virtue of its close proximity, provides better visualization of the mitral valve apparatus. TEE imaging provides an accurate understanding of mitral valve structure, as well as identification of morphologic abnormalities of the mitral valve. TEE permits evaluation of the left atrium, left atrial appendage, atrial septum, and the entire mitral valve apparatus, including the annulus, leaflets, chordae tendineae, papillary muscles, and atrial and ventricular walls. Using a single transverse plane transducer, TEE provides a somewhat restricted number of imaging planes, and assessment of the entire mitral valve apparatus may not be possible in all patients. This limitation is overcome by the biplane probe, which provides tomographic sections through the transverse plane, as well as nearly orthogonal longitudinal planes.[1]

Biplane TEE permits evaluation of both segments of the anterior mitral leaflet (lateral and medial) and of all three scallops of the posterior mitral leaflets (medial, middle, and lateral) by the use of a combination of transgastric short-axis and two-chamber views and of four-chamber, five-chamber, and two-chamber views from the midesophageal position (Table 6-1).

The transgastric short-axis view shows the entire mitral valve and its opening, and it is possible to evaluate both segments of the anterior leaflets and all three scallops of the posterior leaflet (see Ch. 4, Fig. 4-20). The transgastric two-chamber view permits evaluation of the medial scallop of the posterior leaflet and of the lateral segment of the anterior leaflet (see Ch. 4, Fig. 4-30). The four-chamber view with a slight posterior tilt generally permits visualization of the medial segment of the anterior leaflet and of the middle scallop of the posterior leaflet (see Ch. 4, Fig. 4-14). A four-chamber view with slight anterior tilt would generally permit evaluation of the lateral segment of the anterior leaflet and lateral scallop of the posterior leaflet (see Ch. 4, Fig. 4-15). A two-chamber view from the midesophageal position (approximately 30 cm from the incissors) usually displays the lateral segment of the anterior leaflet and medial or middle scallop of the posterior mitral leaflet (see Ch. 4, Fig. 4-27). With the use of these scanning methods,

Table 6-1. TEE Evaluation of Anterior and Posterior Mitral Valve Leaflets

View	Segments of Anterior Mitral Leaflet	Scallops of Posterior Leaflet
Transgastric short-axis	Lateral and medial	Medial, middle, and lateral
Transgastric two-chamber	Lateral	Medial
Four-chamber (posterior tilt)	Medial	Middle
Four-chamber (anterior tilt)	Lateral	Lateral
Two-chamber (midesophageal)	Lateral	Medial or middle

detailed evaluation of the mitral valve, chordae tendineae, papillary muscle, and annulus can be performed. With the use of this type of examination technique, more precise localization of the anatomic fault responsible for mitral regurgitation, including endocarditis, perforation, mitral valve aneurysm, and rupture chordae tendineae with flail leaflet, is feasible.[2] This information regarding the type, cause, and degree of structural abnormality of the various components of the mitral valve apparatus is important to predict the feasibility of mitral valve repair.[3] Quantification of mitral regurgitation would most likely be enhanced by use of the nearly orthogonal views by biplane TEE that permit visual construction of three-dimensional distribution of mitral regurgitation.[1]

MITRAL REGURGITATION

Characteristics of Mitral Regurgitation Jets

Eccentric mitral regurgitation jets are visualized in patients with flail leaflet, severe localized prolapse of one of the scallops caused by elongated and redundant chordae tendineae, and perforation. The eccentric jet is directed opposite to the involved mitral valve leaflet. Lack of leaflet coaptation caused by rheumatic disease, papillary muscle dysfunction, dilated annulus, and dilated cardiomyopathy usually produces more centrally located jets (Figs. 6-1 to 6-3). Systolic anterior motion of the mitral valve in patients with hypertrophic obstructive cardiomyopathy with associated mitral regurgitation produces a regurgitant jet directed posteriorly into the left atrium.

In patients with eccentric regurgitant jets, the jet impacts the receiving chamber wall and results in underestimation of the regurgitation severity. This is because of the *Coanda effect* that results from the jet striking a cardiac chamber wall and losing considerable energy; the resultant jet occupies only a small area, even though the regurgitation is severe.[4] This effect is minimized with the transesophageal approach, probably because of the short ultrasonic beam path and subsequent superior resolution that compensates, to some degree, for the Coanda effect.

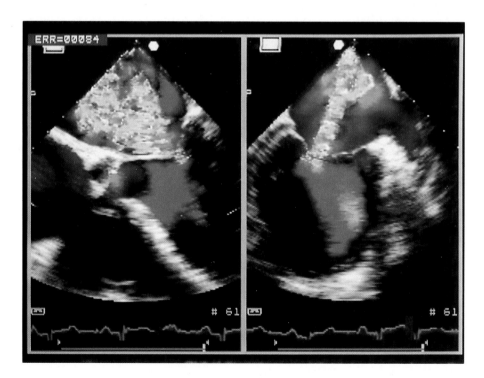

Fig. 6-1. Biplanar study of severe dilated cardiomyopathy and mitral regurgitation. *(Left)* Transverse four-chamber view. *(Right)* Longitudinal two-chamber view. Mitral regurgitation is depicted as a mosaic flow pattern in the left atrium.

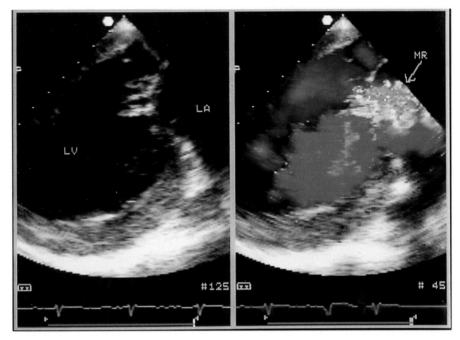

Fig. 6-2. Dilated cardiomyopathy. *(Left)* Transgastric two-chamber view demonstrating an enlarged left ventricle (LV) and global hypokinesis (end-systolic frame). *(Right)* Mitral regurgitation (MR), as seen on color Doppler mapping. LA, left atrium.

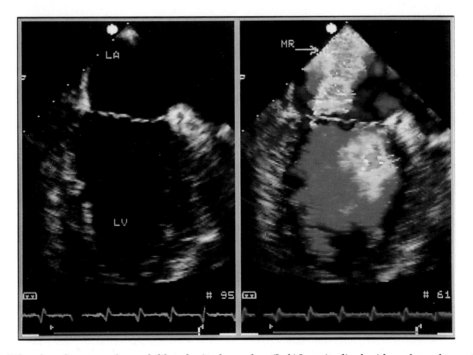

Fig. 6-3. Dilated cardiomyopathy and dilated mitral annulus. *(Left)* Longitudinal midesophageal two-chamber view showing a dilated left ventricle (LV) and left atrium (LA). *(Right)* Moderate mitral regurgitation (MR).

Quantitation of Mitral Regurgitation

Estimates of mitral regurgitation by biplane TEE are semiquantitative. Criteria used to evaluate severity of mitral regurgitation include jet width at the origin, jet length, jet area, and systolic reversal of flow in the pulmonary veins.[5] A recent study[1] assessing mitral regurgitation by biplane TEE found this technique to be highly sensitive in identifying mitral regurgitation and in providing an accurate estimation of its severity. The following criteria were presented for grading the severity of mitral regurgitation as detected by this method: maximum regurgitant jet areas of less than 1.5 cm^2 predicted none to trivial regurgitation, 1.5 to 4 cm^2 predicted mild regurgitation, 4 to 7 cm^2 predicted moderate regurgitation, and more than 7 cm^2 predicted severe regurgitation as compared with angiographic gradings; respective sensitivities and specificities were 88 percent and 94 percent, 82 percent and 95 percent, 100 percent and 95 percent, and 83 percent and 100 percent. These researchers were the first to offer clear criteria for grading the severity of mitral regurgitation on transesophageal scans, but similar investigations from other institutions will be needed to accumulate additional data of this nature.

Consideration should be given to the type of lesion causing regurgitation. Flail mitral valve leaflet and large perforation with eccentric jets should generally result in significant regurgitation. Since the left atrium is foreshortened from transesophageal approach, the ratio of the jet area to the left atrial area is not used for quantitation of the mitral regurgitation.[5]

Retrograde flow into the pulmonary veins during systole (Fig. 6-4) or suppression of the normally prominent systolic pulmonary vein waveform (S-wave)[6] from transesophageal pulsed Doppler of pulmonary venous flow has been noted in our laboratory, and in others, to occur with significant mitral regurgitation[7,8] (Figs. 6-5 and 6-6). This finding is

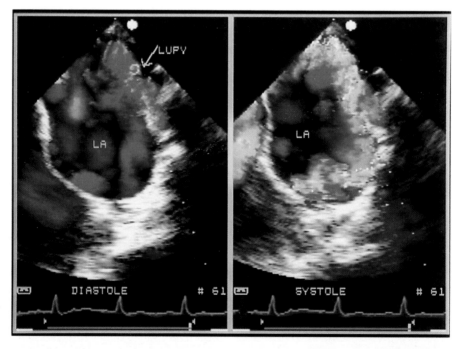

Fig. 6-4. Severe mitral regurgitation producing retrograde regurgitant flow in the left upper pulmonary vein (LUPV). *(Left)* Normal forward flow is depicted in red during left ventricular diastole. *(Right)* Retrograde flow into LUPV is seen as a mosaic of colors during left ventricular systole. LA, left atrium.

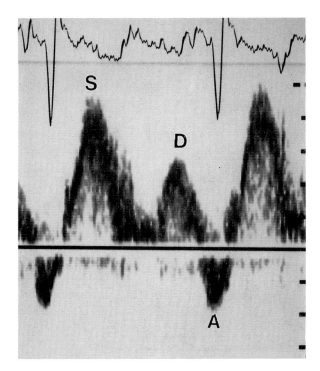

Fig. 6-5. Pulsed Doppler recording of normal pulmonary vein velocity curve. Pulmonary vein velocity consists of retrograde velocity at atrial contraction (A), followed by systolic forward flow (S) and diastolic forward flow (D).

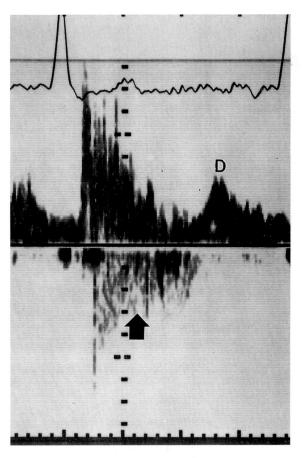

Fig. 6-6. Reversal of systolic flow (arrow) in a patient with severe mitral regurgitation. D, diastolic forward flow.

particularly important in patients with eccentric regurgitant jets, as discussed above, in whom the regurgitation severity may appear mild when in fact it is moderate or severe.

Mitral Regurgitation of Normal Valves

Mitral regurgitant flow patterns have been documented with precordial Doppler flow imaging in healthy persons, but with a predominance of right-sided valve regurgitation.[9-11] The incidence of this physiologic backflow in apparently normal mitral valves varies widely from 0 to 40 percent.[9] Comparisons of transthoracic and transesophageal color Doppler imaging reveal a fourfold higher sensitivity of the transesophageal technique in the detection of a regurgitant flow over the mitral valve.[12]

Transesophageal color Doppler imaging usually reveals a specific color pattern of holosystolic mild mitral regurgitation. These patients have a normal mitral valve apparatus, normal left ventricular size, and normal wall motion.

MITRAL VALVE PROLAPSE

Biplane imaging gives an accurate understanding of mitral valve prolapse by depicting the part of the posterior leaflet (medial, middle, and lateral scallop) and anterior leaflet (lateral and medial) that is pro-

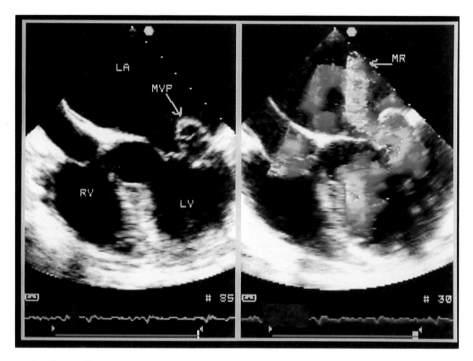

Fig. 6-7. Mitral valve prolapse (MVP). *(Left)* Transverse four-chamber view showing prolapse of the posterior mitral valve leaflet. *(Right)* Mitral regurgitation (MR). LA, left atrium; LV, left ventricle; RV, right ventricle.

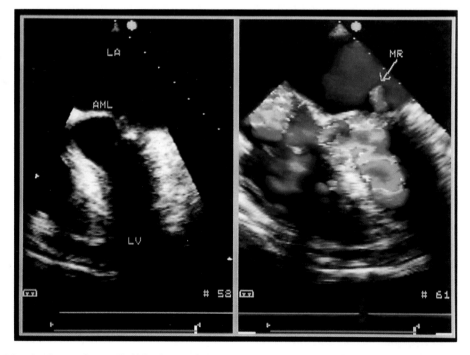

Fig. 6-8. Mitral valve prolapse. *(Left)* Prolapse of the anterior mitral valve leaflet (AML). *(Right)* Minimal mitral regurgitation (MR). LA, left atrium; LV, left ventricle.

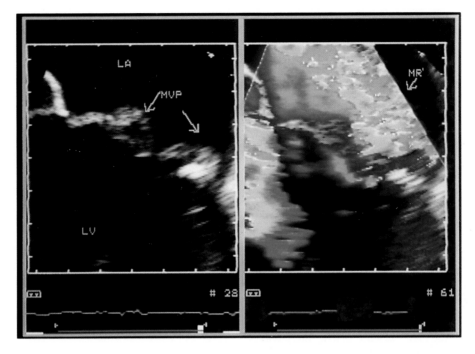

Fig. 6-9. Magnified view of the mitral valve in patient with mitral valve prolapse (MVP). *(Left)* Thickened and redundant anterior and posterior leaflets. *(Right)* Severe mitral regurgitation (MR). LA, left atrium; LV, left ventricle.

lapsing. Thus, the pathologic configuration of mitral valve prolapse can be understood precisely and accurately. This is important when surgical repairs are to be undertaken in mitral regurgitation because of complications of mitral valve prolapse. This knowledge is important for planning the method of repair and for assessing the competency of a valve after the repairs are made (see Ch. 16).

The TEE findings of mitral valve prolapse include a circular or coil cusp or whiplike protrusion of a scallop of the posterior leaflet (Fig. 6-7) or segment of the anterior leaflet into the left atrium in systole[13] (Fig. 6-8). Color Doppler mapping identifies the presence of mitral regurgitation and provides an accurate estimation of its severity. Prolapse of the posterior mitral valve leaflet produces a regurgitant jet directed anteriorly and a prolapse of the anterior mitral valve leaflet produces a regurgitant jet directed posteriorly.

TEE is also useful in assessing the thickness of the mitral leaflet and evaluating for valve redundancy (Fig. 6-9).

RUPTURED CHORDAE TENDINEAE

TEE is superior to TTE in the diagnosis of ruptured chordae tendineae.[14] A recent study[15] found TTE detection of ruptured chordae tendineae to have a sensitivity of 35 percent and a specificity of 100 percent. The sensitivity of TEE in the detection of ruptured chordae tendineae was 100 percent, and the specificity was 100 percent. TEE findings of ruptured chordae tendineae include abnormal systolic echo in the left atrium, which is associated with significant mitral regurgitation (Figs. 6-10 to 6-14). The mitral regurgitant jet is usually eccentric and directed opposite to the flail mitral leaflet. Other signs of severe mitral regurgitation include systolic reversal of flow in the

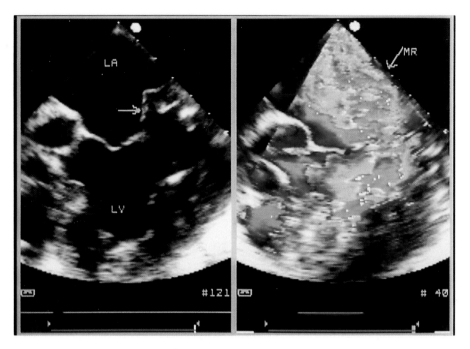

Fig. 6-10. Ruptured chordae tendineae. *(Left)* Transverse midesophageal plane showing a flail posterior mitral leaflet (arrow). *(Right)* Severe mitral regurgitation (MR). LA, left atrium; LV, left ventricle.

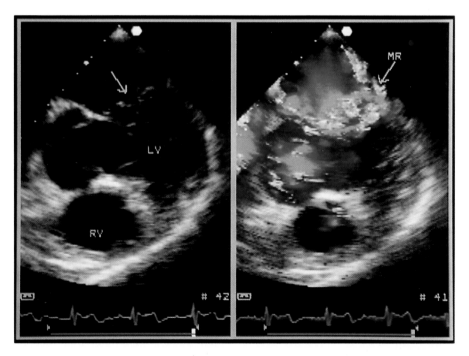

Fig. 6-11. *(Left)* Ruptured chordae tendineae to posterior mitral leaflet (arrow). *(Right)* Color Doppler mapping demonstrating an eccentric mitral regurgitant (MR) jet. LV, left ventricle; RV, right ventricle.

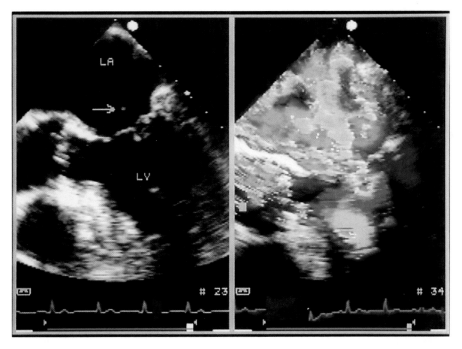

Fig. 6-12. Ruptured chordae tendineae to posterior mitral leaflet. *(Left)* Abnormal systolic echo (arrow) in left atrium (LA) representing chordal structure. *(Right)* Severe mitral regurgitation. The regurgitant jet occupies the entire left atrial cavity. LV, left ventricle.

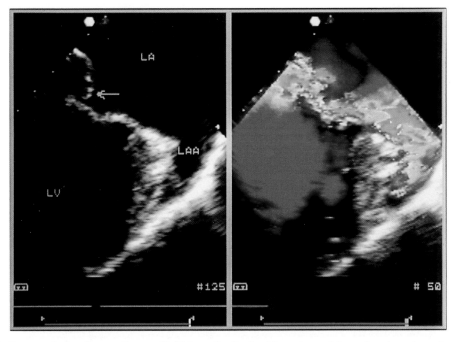

Fig. 6-13. Ruptured chordae tendineae. *(Left)* Longitudinal midesophageal two-chamber view showing a flail posterior mitral leaflet (arrow). *(Right)* Eccentric mitral regurgitant jet directed to the left atrial appendage (LAA). LA, left atrium; LV, left ventricle.

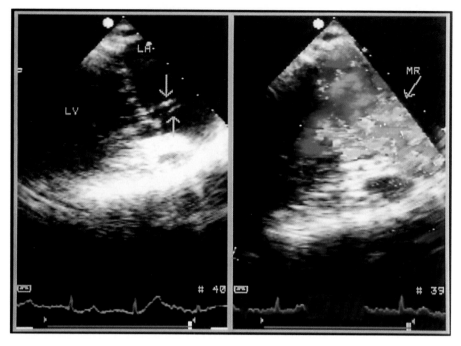

Fig. 6-14. Ruptured chordae tendineae to anterior mitral leaflet. *(Left)* Two-chamber trangastric view demonstrating chordal structures (arrows) in the left atrium (LA). *(Right)* Severe mitral regurgitation (MR). LV, left ventricle.

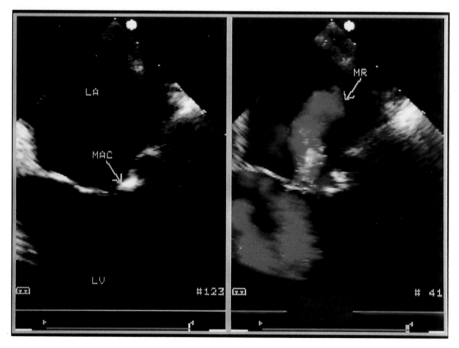

Fig. 6-15. *(Left)* Transverse midesophageal view showing posterior mitral annulus calcification (MAC). *(Right)* Mild mitral regurgitation (MR). LA, left atrium; LV, left ventricle.

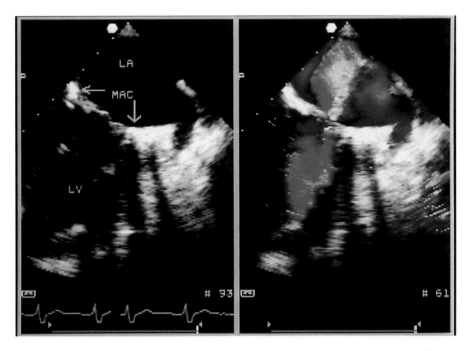

Fig. 6-16. *(Left)* Longitudinal midesophageal two-chamber view in patient with anterior and posterior mitral annulus calcification (MAC). *(Right)* Mild mitral regurgitation. LA, left atrium; LV, left ventricle.

pulmonary veins (Figs. 6-4 to 6-6) and a wide mitral regurgitant jet at its origin.

MITRAL ANNULUS CALCIFICATION

TTE is particularly limited in the evaluation of mitral regurgitation in patients with mitral annulus calcification and in those with scarring and calcification of the leaflets. It is possible to underestimate grossly the degree of mitral regurgitation in this patient subgroup. TEE is much more sensitive and accurate in detecting and quantifying mitral regurgitation in these patients (Figs. 6-15 and 6-16). Furthermore, subvalvular disease can be assessed much more accurately.

ISCHEMIC MITRAL REGURGITATION

In ischemic mitral regurgitation, the valve may show prolapse but frequently appears normal.[16] Most patients in this category show posterior papillary muscle dysfunction, which is best assessed using the transgastric short axis view at the level of the papillary muscle (Figs. 6-17 and 6-18).

TEE has also been safely used in the evaluation of patients with acute myocardial infarction complicated by papillary muscle rupture or ventricular septal rupture, especially in patients with suboptimal and nondiagnostic thoracic images.[17-19] Biplane imaging is also useful in differentiating ventricular septal rupture from papillary muscle rupture.

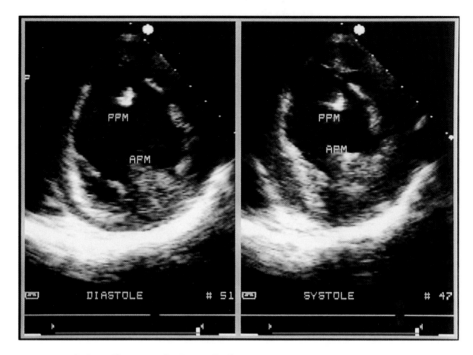

Fig. 6-17. Posteromedial papillary muscle (PPM) dysfunction in patient with posterior wall infarction. *(Left)* The PPM is highly echogenic as a result of scarring. *(Right)* Impaired contractility of PPM. APM, anterior papillary muscle.

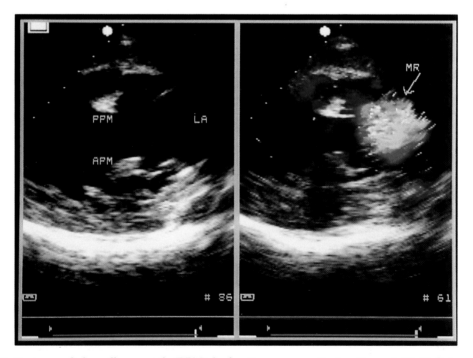

Fig. 6-18. Posteromedial papillary muscle (PPM) dysfunction; same patient as Figure 6-17. *(Left)* Longitudinal transgastric two-chamber view showing signs of scarring of PPM. *(Right)* Moderate mitral regurgitation (MR). APM, anterior papillary muscle; LA, left atrium.

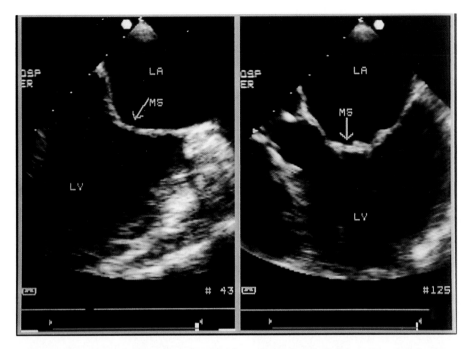

Fig. 6-19. Mitral stenosis (MS). *(Left)* Longitudinal midesophageal two-chamber view. *(Right)* Transverse four-chamber view. The mitral valve is thickened and domes in diastole. LA, left atrium; LV, left ventricle.

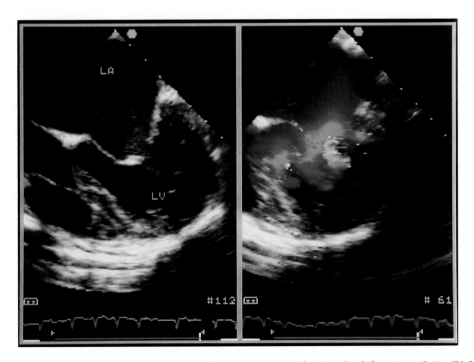

Fig. 6-20. Mitral stenosis. *(Left)* Spontaneous echo contrast is evident in the left atrium (LA). *(Right)* Color Doppler image during diastole showing turbulence at level of mitral valve. LV, left ventricle.

MITRAL STENOSIS

In patients with mitral stenosis, TTE using continuous-wave Doppler techniques provides information regarding the mean and end-diastolic gradients and mitral valve area in the majority of patients.[20] Currently, most esophageal probes have the capability of steerable, continuous-wave Doppler, which permits accurate calculation of mitral valve area, using the midesophageal four-chamber view (Fig. 6-19). TEE is far superior to TTE, however, in detecting spontaneous echo contrast in the left atrial cavity (Fig. 6-20) and in evaluating appendage and body thrombi.[20-23] TEE also provides better evaluation of leaflet mobility, thickness, location, and extent of calcification in the body of the leaflet or commissures, as well as the degree of involvement of chordae tendineae and subvalvular mitral apparatus. This information is of value in predicting the feasibility of balloon mitral valvuloplasty or open mitral commissurotomy.[24,25]

In candidates for balloon mitral valvuloplasty, precatheterization TEE may detect unsuspected left atrial thrombi.[26] During mitral valvuloplasty, TEE has been demonstrated to be helpful in guiding transseptal puncture; in assessing the extent of postdilation mitral regurgitation; or in detecting catheter complications, such as myocardial perforation and pericardial effusion. Furthermore, the presence of interatrial shunting can be readily assessed at the end of the procedure, making cineangiography of the left ventricle and left atrium not necessary (see Fig. 6-21).

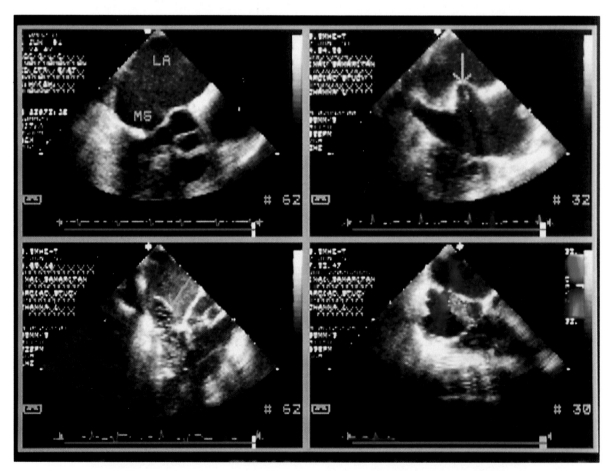

Fig. 6-21. Mitral balloon valvuloplasty. *(Upper left)* Mitral stenosis (MS), dilated left atrium (LA), and spontaneous echo contrast. *(Upper right)* Transseptal puncture (arrow). *(Lower left)* Balloon inflated (arrow). Note increase in spontaneous echo contrast. *(Lower right)* Small residual atrial septal defect with a left-to-right shunt following the procedure.

Because of the potential risk of embolization, we recommend that TEE be performed in all candidates for balloon mitral valvuloplasty.

REFERENCES

1. Yoshida K, Yoshikawa J, Yamaura Y, et al. Assessment of mitral regurgitation by biplane transesophageal color Doppler flow mapping. Circulation 1990; 82:1121–1126.
2. Schlüter M, Kremer P, Hanrath P. Transesophageal 2-D echocardiographic feature of flail mitral leaflet due to ruptured chordae tendineae. Am Heart J 1984; 108:609–610.
3. Carpentier A. Cardiac valve surgery—the "French correction." J Thorac Cardiovasc Surg 1983; 86:323–337.
4. Chen C, Thomas JD, Anconina J, et al. Impact of impinging wall jet on color Doppler quantification of mitral regurgitation. Circulation 1991; 84:712–720.
5. Kleinman JP, Czer LSC, DeRobertis M, et al. A quantitative comparison of transesophageal and epicardial color Doppler echocardiography in the intraoperative assessment of mitral regurgitation. Am J Cardiol 1989; 64:1168–1172.
6. Kuecherer HF, Muhiudeen IA, Kusumoto FM, et al. Estimation of mean left atrial pressure from transesophageal pulsed Doppler echocardiography of pulmonary venous flow. Circulation 1990; 82:1127–1139.
7. Jain S, Moos S, Awad M, et al. Assessment of mitral regurgitation severity using pulmonary venous flow by transesophageal color Doppler. Circulation 1989; 80:571 (abst).
8. Pearson AC, Castello R, Wallace PM, Labovitz AJ. Effect of mitral regurgitation on pulmonary venous velocities derived by transesophageal echocardiography. Circulation 1989; 80:571 (abst).
9. Kostucki W, Vandenbossche JL, Friart A, Englert M. Pulsed Doppler regurgitant flow patterns of normal valves. Am J Cardiol 1986; 58:309–313.
10. Come PC, Riley MF, Carl LV, Nakao S. Pulsed Doppler echocardiographic evaluation of valvular regurgitation in patients with mitral valve prolapse: comparison with normal subjects. J Am Coll Cardiol 1986; 8:1355–1364.
11. Abbasi AS, Allen MW, DeCristofaro D, Ungar I. Detection and estimation of the degree of mitral regurgitation by range-gated pulsed Doppler echocardiography. Circulation 1980; 61:143–147.
12. Taams MA, Gussenhoven EJ, Cahalan MK, et al. Transesophageal Doppler color flow imaging in the detection of native and Björk-Shiley mitral valve regurgitation. J Am Coll Cardiol 1989; 13:95–99.
13. Joh Y, Yoshikawa J, Yoshida K, et al. Transesophageal echocardiographic findings of mitral valve prolapse. J of Cardiol 1989; 19:85–95.
14. Schlüter M, Kremer P, Hanrath P. Transesophageal 2-D echocardiographic feature of flail mitral leaflet due to ruptured chordae tendineae. Am Heart J 1984; 108:609–610.
15. Hozumi T, Yoshikawa J, Yoshida K, et al. Direct visualization of ruptured chordae tendineae by transesophageal two-dimensional echocardiography, J Am Coll Cardiol 1990; 16:1315–1319.
16. Sheikh KH, Bengtson JR, Rankin JC, et al. Intraoperative transesophageal Doppler color flow imaging used to guide patient selection and operative treatment of ischemic mitral regurgitation. Circulation 1991; 84:594–604.
17. Koenig K, Kasper W, Hofmann T, et al. Transesophageal echocardiography for diagnosis of rupture of the ventricular septum or left ventricular papillary muscle during acute myocardial infarction. Am J Cardiol 1987; 59:362.
18. Oh JK, Seward JB, Khandheria BK. Transesophageal echocardiography in the intensive care unit. Circulation 1988; 78:298 (abst).
19. Patel AM, Miller FA, Khandheria BK, et al. Role of the transesophageal echocardiography in the diagnosis of papillary muscle rupture secondary to myocardial infarction. Am Heart J 1989; 118:1330–1333.
20. Bansal RC, Shah PM. Usefulness of echo-Doppler in management of patients with valvular heart disease. Curr Probl Cardiol 1989; 14:282–350.
21. Daniel WG, Nellessen U, Schroder E, et al. Left atrial spontaneous echo contrast in mitral valve disease: an indicator for an increased thromboembolic risk. J Am Coll Cardiol 1988; 11:1204–1211.
22. Bansal RC, Heywood JT, Applegate PM, Jutzy KR. Detection of left atrial thrombi by two-dimensional echocardiography and surgical correlation in 148 patients with mitral valve disease. Am J Cardiol 1989; 64:243–246.
23. Herzog CA, Bass D, Kane M, Asinger R. Two-dimensional echocardiographic imaging of left atrial appendage thrombi. J Am Coll Cardiol 1984; 3:1340–1344.
24. Reid CL, Chandraratna AN, Kawanishi DT, et al. Influence of mitral valve morphology on double-balloon catheter balloon valvuloplasty in patients with mitral stenosis. Circulation 1989; 80:515–524.
25. Kronzon I, Tunick PA, Schwinger ME, et al. Transesophageal echocardiography during percutaneous mitral valvuloplasty. J Am Soc Echocardiol 1989; 2:380–385.
26. Kronzon I, Tunick PA, Glassman E, et al. Transesophageal echocardiography to detect atrial clots in candidates for percutaneous transseptal mitral balloon valvuloplasty. J Am Coll Cardiol 1990; 16:1320–1322.

7 Evaluation of the Tricuspid and Pulmonary Valves

TRICUSPID VALVE

The tricuspid valve leaflets can be imaged using both the horizontal and the longitudinal planes. Four-chamber and right ventricular inflow views obtained by transverse single-plane transesophageal imaging permit evaluation of the tricuspid valve, right atrium, and right ventricle. The superior vena cava and atrial septum are best seen by obtaining the basal views with the biplane probe.

TRICUSPID VALVE REGURGITATION

The etiology of tricuspid regurgitation, including annular dilation, vegetation, perforation, flail leaflet, and rheumatic and carcinoid disease, can be evaluated. The degree of tricuspid regurgitation is roughly semiquantitated using the area of the regurgitant jet similar to the transthoracic approach (Figs. 7-1 and 7-2). The addition of continuous-wave Doppler to the esophageal probe permits accurate determination of transvalvular pressure gradient and calculation of pulmonary artery systolic pressure (Fig. 7-3).

PULMONARY VALVE

The pulmonary valve is an anteriorly situated structure that is generally well imaged by transthoracic echocardiography (TTE). The use of TEE with a transverse imaging probe provides an image of the main pulmonary artery and its bifurcation along with the right pulmonary artery branch (see Ch. 4, Fig. 4-5). The right ventricular outflow tract, pulmonary valve, main pulmonary artery, and contiguous anatomy are also optimally visualized in the longitudinal scanning plane (see Ch. 4, Figs. 4-22 and 4-23). Visualization of the distal portion of both right and left pulmonary arteries is enhanced with longitudinal imaging.

TTE is generally satisfactory for evaluating the presence and severity of pulmonic stenosis and regurgitation. TEE using biplane imaging is likely to prove superior in the evaluation of the right ventricular outflow tract, the pulmonary artery, and its branches (Fig. 7-4). It may provide useful information regarding infundibular stenosis (Fig. 7-5), hypoplasia, and atresia of the pulmonary arteries, and peripheral pulmonary arterial stenosis.

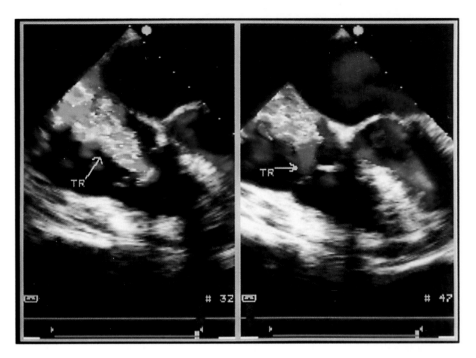

Fig. 7-1. Transverse four-chamber view of tricuspid regurgitation (TR). *(Left)* Moderate TR in patient with pulmonary hypertension. *(Right)* Mild to moderate TR following a right ventricular infarction.

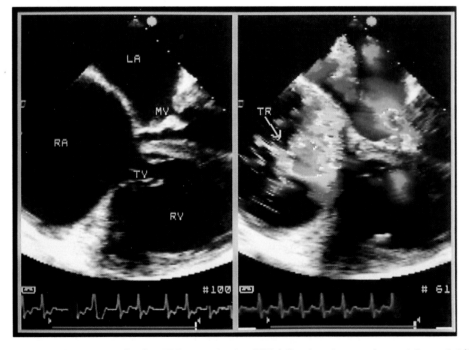

Fig. 7-2. Severe residual tricuspid valve (TV) regurgitation (TR) following closure of an atrial septal defect. *(Left)* Transverse four-chamber view showing an enlarged right atrium (RA) and right ventricle (RV). The mitral valve (MV) is thickened and redundant. *(Right)* Color Doppler image demonstrating severe tricuspid regurgitation.

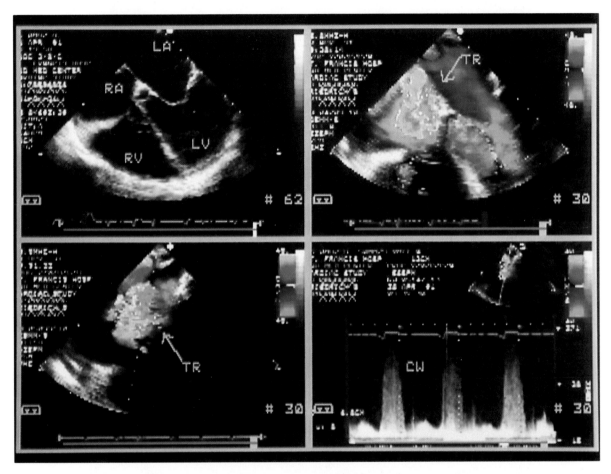

Fig. 7-3. Severe tricuspid regurgitation (TR) in patient with dilated cardiomyopathy and pulmonary hypertension. *(Upper left)* All four cardiac chambers are dilated. *(Upper right)* Severe TR is seen as a mosaic of blue and yellow. *(Lower left)* Transverse plane at coronary sinus depicting severe TR. This view permits accurate velocity measurement of the regurgitant velocity for determination of pulmonary artery systolic pressure. *(Lower right)* Continuous-wave (CW) Doppler spectral recording of maximum regurgitant velocity. The pulmonary artery systolic pressure was calculated at 60 mmHg. LA, left atrium; LV, left ventricle; RA, right atrium; RV, right ventricle.

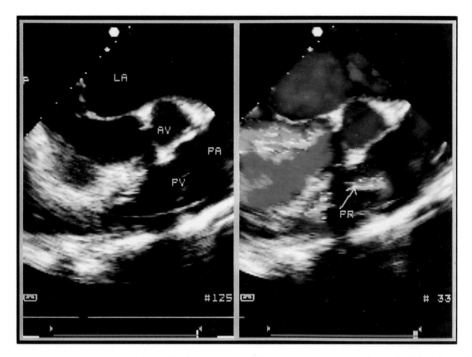

Fig. 7-4. Pulmonary valve regurgitation (PR). *(Left)* Longitudinal basal view demonstrating the pulmonary valve (PV) and main pulmonary artery (PA). The linear echo-dense structure in the right ventricular outflow is a Swan-Ganz catheter. *(Right)* Color Doppler mapping reveals mild PR. AV, aortic valve; LA, left atrium.

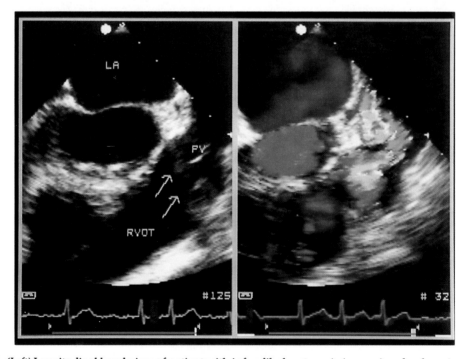

Fig. 7-5. *(Left)* Longitudinal basal view of patient with infundibular stenosis (arrows) and pulmonic valve (PV) stenosis. *(Right)* Turbulent flow is noted in the proximal main pulmonary artery. LA, left atrium; RVOT, right ventricular outflow tract.

8 Prosthetic Valve Evaluation and Recognition of Dysfunction

Despite improvements in valve design and surgical technique, prosthetic valve dysfunction continues to be a common problem. Prosthetic valves are subject to the development of various complications, including severe stenosis, regurgitation, endocarditis, thromboembolism, hemolysis, and bleeding from anticoagulant therapy. Clinical examination is inexact and is often confounded by superimposed cardiovascular problems, such as ventricular dysfunction, multivalvular disease, and ischemic heart disease.

Over the years, fluoroscopy, phonocardiography, and echocardiography have assisted in the serial noninvasive evaluation of prosthetic valve function.[1-3] All patients with prosthetic cardiac valves should have a comprehensive 2-D Doppler echocardiographic and color Doppler examination that will serve as a baseline study to compare with future examinations when there is suspected prosthetic valve dysfunction. Normal Doppler-derived values for pressure and flow gradients are now available for most prosthetic valves.[4,5] Two-dimensional echocardiography has been useful in the assessment of left ventricular function, calcification of the bioprosthetic valves, large vegetations, and rocking motion noted with dehiscence of the ring. The introduction of continuous-wave Doppler echocardiography has been extremely useful in the assessment of obstruction across the various types of prosthetic valves.[6,7] Complete continuous-wave Doppler examination using multiple precordial windows is useful in the accurate measurement of mean gradient across the prosthetic heart valves.[7] Prosthetic aortic and mitral valve areas can also be calculated using continuity equation and pressure half-time methods, respectively.[8] The mechanism and cause of prosthetic valve obstruction (e.g., tissue ingrowth, thrombus or vegetation) are better assessed, however, by TEE.

FLOW MASKING

The metal components of the prosthetic valve act as strong reflectors of ultrasound and reflect a great deal of ultrasound energy back to the transducer, making ultrasound penetration behind the prosthesis very difficult. These devices also create strong reverberations behind the prosthesis. Thus, the flow behind the prosthesis cannot be accurately evaluated because of the phenomenon of *flow masking*, which is the result of poor ultrasound penetration behind the prosthetic valve, and reverberation artifacts (Fig. 8-1). From the transthoracic approach, apical views are generally suitable for assessment of prosthetic mitral and tricuspid stenosis because the Doppler

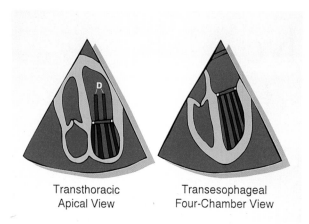

Transthoracic Apical View

Transesophageal Four-Chamber View

Fig. 8-1. Flow masking caused by a St. Jude mitral valve prosthesis. Masking of the left atrium occurs from the transthoracic apical four-chamber view. Masking of the left ventricle occurs from the transesophageal approach. D, disks.

beam traverses the stenotic jets without interference from the prosthetic valve. For assessment of prosthetic aortic stenosis, however, it is best to interrogate from multiple positions, including right parasternal, suprasternal, and apical. From the apical position alone, it may be possible to mask the jet of aortic stenosis because of flow masking from the poppet in the ascending aorta.

A major limitation of TTE is in the evaluation of prosthetic valve regurgitation. For prosthetic mitral and tricuspid regurgitation, apical and parasternal windows may be unrewarding because both left and right atrial cavities are obscured by the flow-masking phenomenon and reverberation artifacts. The presence of an aortic prosthesis also obscures the left atrial cavity. The apical and parasternal views are generally suitable for assessment of prosthetic aortic regurgitation, because there is no significant interference in the left ventricular outflow tract from the prosthetic aortic valve. A localized region of flow masking is generally seen in the left ventricular outflow tract just below the prosthetic aortic ring. After complete continuous-wave Doppler examination using multiple transducer positions, it is generally possible to suspect prosthetic mitral regurgitation, but precise quantitation is often difficult and inaccurate. TEE provides a clear view of the left atrial cavity

without interference from the prosthetic valve (Fig. 8-1) and is extremely useful in the assessment of spontaneous echo contrast, thrombus, vegetations, and the presence and severity of prosthetic mitral regurgitation.[10-13] This technique permits a clear distinction between central and perivalvular prosthetic mitral regurgitation jets. Semiquantification of the regurgitation is performed by using the jet area, length, and width at its origin (discussed in Ch. 6). The left atrium is often foreshortened in the transesophageal examination, and the jet area to left atrial area ratios are not used. Perivalvular regurgitation jets are often eccentric, and biplane TEE is more helpful in precise localization and better quantitation of these leaks. Single plane TEE is not as useful in the assessment of prosthetic aortic regurgitation, as the ultrasonic beam has to first traverse the prosthetic aortic valve, thereby creating flow masking in the left ventricular outflow tract. However, we have observed a significant improvement in assessment of prosthetic aortic regurgitation with the use of biplane TEE. TEE is extremely useful in the evaluation of complications of endocarditis, such as vegetations, ring abscesses, flail bioprosthetic cusps, sewing ring dehiscence, and perivalvular regurgitation (see Ch. 10).

EVALUATION OF MITRAL VALVE PROSTHESES

Normal Prosthetic Valves

All prosthetic valves have a trivial amount of physiologic regurgitation, referred to as closing volume. This closure or backflow-related mitral regurgitation is seen as a transient, low-velocity, pure red flow in the left atrium in early systole at the time of the closure of the prosthetic valve[12] (Fig. 8-2). The physiologic jet is less than 2 cm long and 1 cm wide, originating from the valve leaflets or poppets, and has been reported in 35 percent of mitral valves by TEE but only in 8 percent by TTE.[14] Recognition of this normal finding is important in avoiding misinterpretation of this retrograde flow as signifying pathology.

Tissue valves usually have a single central jet of physiologic regurgitation (Fig. 8-3), whereas mechanical valves may have multiple jets, depending on their type and number of inflow orifices. In the presence of

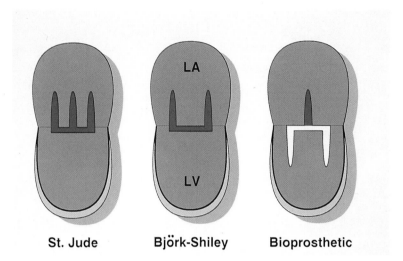

St. Jude   Björk-Shiley   Bioprosthetic

Fig. 8-2. Diagram showing physiologic mitral regurgitation with transesophageal color Doppler echocardiography in three prosthetic mitral valves. LA, left atrium; LV, left ventricle.

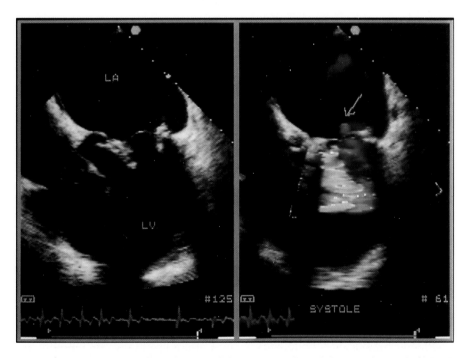

Fig. 8-3. Transverse four-chamber view of a normal Carpentier-Edwards bioprosthesis. *(Left)* The bioprosthetic leaflets are thin and pliable and normally bulge toward the left atrium (LA) during systole. *(Right)* Color Doppler showing minimal physiologic mitral regurgitation (arrow). LV, left ventricle.

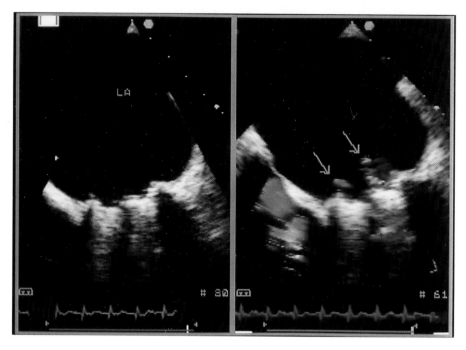

Fig. 8-4. Normal functioning Björk-Shiley mitral prosthesis. *(Left)* Magnified transverse four-chamber view; systolic frame. *(Right)* Color Doppler showing two identical jets (arrows) that represent physiologic regurgitation. LA, left atrium.

a normal-functioning Björk-Shiley mitral valve prosthesis, transesophageal color Doppler mapping reveals two identical jets representing blood volume necessary to close the disk and blood volume passing the disk and housing during systole (Fig. 8-4). One discrete central and a couple of peripheral jets of mitral regurgitation are commonly visualized with a normally-functioning Medtronic-Hall mitral prosthesis. It is common to see several peripheral and a single, small, narrow, central mitral regurgitation jet with a normally functioning St. Jude prosthesis[13] (Figs. 8-5 and 8-6). A mild degree of swirling or spontaneous echo contrast in the left atrium is noted with most prostheses, especially with an enlarged left atrium and atrial fibrillation. Significant spontaneous echo contrast in the left atrium is, however, abnormal and may indicate a prethrombotic stage and high embolic potential[15] (Fig. 8-7).

Prosthetic Valve Dysfunction

Several studies reported in the literature have shown that, in patients with suspected mitral prosthetic dysfunction, TEE can provide important information beyond that obtainable from the transthoracic approach.[10–14] Major advantages of TEE include high sensitivity (approximately 100 percent) of color Doppler in the detection and semiquantitation of mitral prosthetic regurgitation; differentiation between paravalvular and central regurgitation[12]; and detection of complications of mitral prosthetic endocarditis, such as abscesses, vegetations, and flail cusps.[16] In our experience, as well as in others, TEE provides new and relevant information that has direct impact on clinical management in approximately 45 to 50 percent of mitral prosthetic valve patients referred with suspected dysfunction.[11,17] Even in patients in

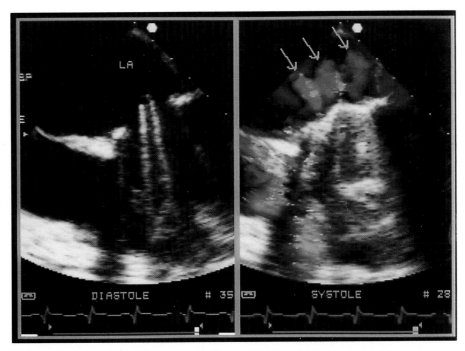

Fig. 8-5. *(Left)* Diastolic frame of transverse four-chamber view of a normal St. Jude mitral valve prosthesis. This view shows both disks in open position aligned parallel to each other. *(Right)* Systolic frame demonstrating three narrow red jets (arrows) of mitral regurgitation; a normal finding on TEE. LA, left atrium.

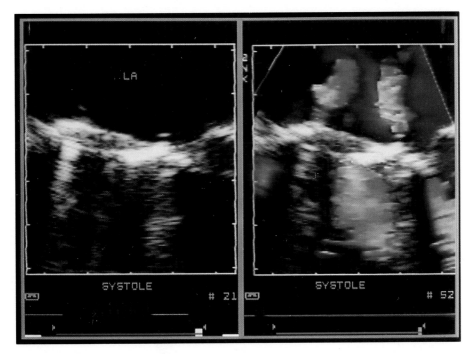

Fig. 8-6. *(Left)* Systolic frame of a normal St. Jude mitral valve prosthesis. *(Right)* Color Doppler showing two peripheral and one discrete central regurgitant jets. LA, left atrium.

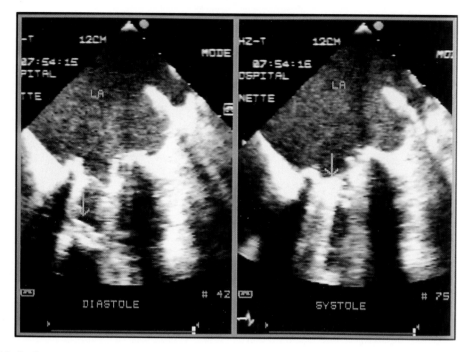

Fig. 8-7. Marked spontaneous echo contrast in left atrium (LA) in patient with history of stroke and Björk-Shiley mitral valve prosthesis. The arrow points to the disk in the open position (diastole) and in the closed position (systole).

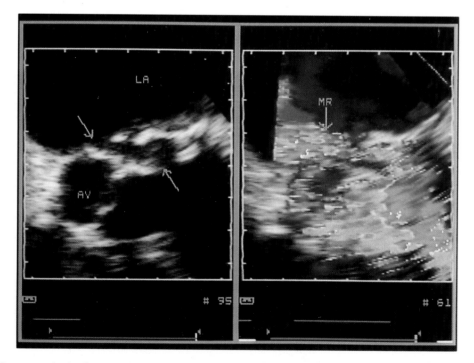

Fig. 8-8. Severe perivalvular regurgitation in patient with a St. Jude mitral valve prosthesis. *(Left)* Magnified transverse view showing area of dehiscence (arrows). *(Right)* Color Doppler image showing an eccentric jet of perivalvular mitral regurgitation (MR). AV, aortic valve; LA, left atrium.

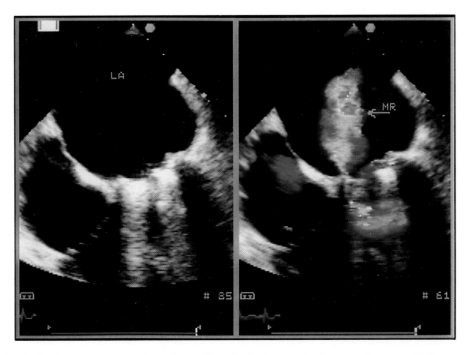

Fig. 8-9. Perivalvular regurgitation in patient with a St. Jude mitral valve prosthesis. *(Left)* Systolic frame in transverse four-chamber view. *(Right)* Color Doppler image showing perivalvular mitral regurgitation (MR). LA, left atrium.

whom the TTE/Doppler examination gave an abnormal result, TEE provided superior definition of the specific abnormality.

TEE is useful in identifying the site of regurgitation.[14] Paravalvular regurgitation with visualization of a defect in the attachment of the ring to the annulus and the associated regurgitant jet in this region can be clearly defined by TEE (Figs. 8-8 and 8-9). It must be understood, however, that the degree of regurgitation in this setting may be underestimated, since the jets are usually eccentric striking the atrial wall, (the *Coanda effect* (see Ch. 6). Central regurgitant jets that can occur with mechanical and biologic prosthetic valves can easily be identified and the regurgitant jet tends to be more central which facilitates quantification.

TEE also has an important role in identifying potential sources of emboli in patients with mitral valve prostheses. TEE can locate the source of an emboli in patients with left atrial or left atrial appendage thrombi. This is in contrast to a much lower yield from TTE. However, TEE may fail to recognize a small thrombus on the sewing ring and on the ventricular surface of the prosthesis.[11] Biplane imaging can potentially improve the diagnostic yield for small thrombi localized on the surface of the sewing ring.

EVALUATION OF AORTIC VALVE PROSTHESES

In aortic prosthesis, the transesophageal approach delineates the extent or absence of prosthetic motion and the presence and severity of regurgitant lesions (Figs. 8-10 and 8-11). The transthoracic approach remains superior to the transesophageal approach in the assessment of aortic prosthetic regurgitation in patients with heavily calcified mitral annuli or from an additional mitral prosthesis. The calcification or mitral prosthesis attenuates the ultrasound beam and results in suboptimal visualization of the regurgitant

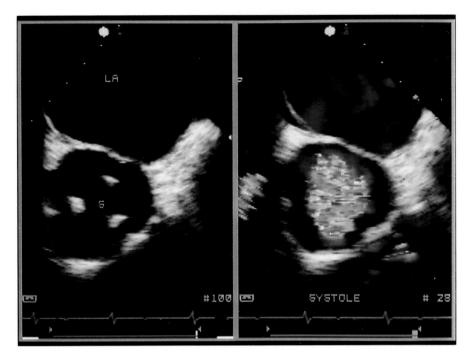

Fig. 8-10. *(Left)* Transverse basal short-axis view of a normal bioprosthetic aortic valve. The three struts (S) are well seen. *(Right)* Color Doppler image showing turbulent flow in the aorta during systole. LA, left atrium.

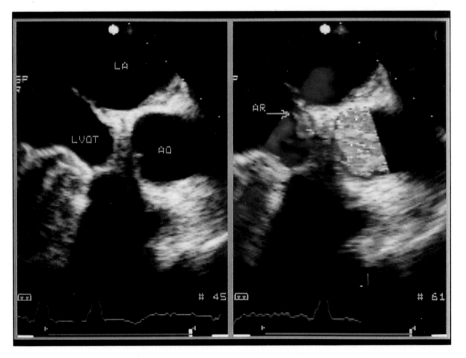

Fig. 8-11. Normal-functioning St. Jude aortic prosthesis. *(Left)* Longitudinal view of left ventricular outflow tract (LVOT) and ascending aorta (AO). *(Right)* Color Doppler map showing minimal physiologic aortic regurgitation (AR). LA, left atrium.

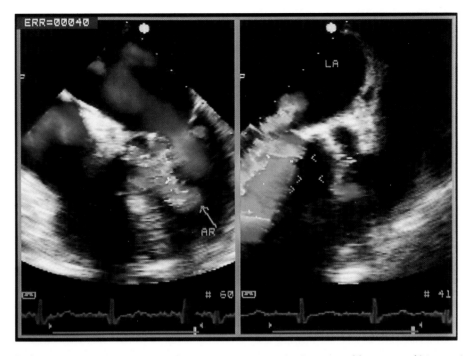

Fig. 8-12. Biplane imaging in a patient with severe aortic regurgitation caused by a tear of bioprosthetic aortic valve leaflet. *(Left)* Transverse five-chamber view demonstrating severe aortic regurgitation (AR) on color Doppler imaging. *(Right)* Longitudinal plane of the left ventricular outflow tract fails to visualize the regurgitant jet due to flow masking (small arrows) caused by the valve struts and prosthetic aortic ring. LA, left atrium.

signals in the left ventricular outflow tract. In some instances, flow masking is marked, and the regurgitant color Doppler signals in the proximal left ventricular outflow tract are almost completely obscured, making estimation of their proximal width, hence the severity of the regurgitant aortic valve jet, difficult (Fig. 8-12). Biplane TEE can be superior, however, in selected patients undergoing difficult transthoracic studies. We have found it useful in cases of suspected prosthetic endocarditis and especially in detecting lesions, such as ring abscesses, vegetations, sinus of valsalva aneurysms, and mitral-aortic intervalvular fibrosa rupture seen with infective endocarditis.

Prosthetic aortic valve stenosis is generally best evaluated from the transthoracic approach, using continuous-wave Doppler from multiple precordial windows. The use of the transesophageal transgastric long-axis view with anteflexion of the tip optimizes visualization of the aortic valve and left ventricular

outflow in long axis. This view best permit continuous-wave Doppler assessment of prosthetic aortic valve stenosis and regurgitation.

EVALUATION OF TRICUSPID VALVE PROSTHESES

There are very few data concerning the usefulness of TEE in the evaluation of tricuspid prostheses.[14] However, one would expect it to be superior to the transthoracic approach in the assessment of tricuspid regurgitation as well as in outlining any vegetations or thrombi involving the prosthesis. A major advantage of the newer transesophageal probes is the addition of continuous-wave Doppler capability, which makes it feasible to measure pressure gradients across obstructed prostheses. It appears that benefits similar to those seen in examining mitral prosthetic valves are likely.

REFERENCES

1. Sands MJ, Lachman AS, O'Reilly DJ, et al. Diagnostic valve of cinefluoroscopy in the evaluation of prosthetic heart valve dysfunction. Am Heart J 1982; 104:622–627.
2. Kotler MN, Segal BL, Parary WR. Echocardiographic and phonocardiographic evaluation of prosthetic heart valves. Cardiovasc Clin 1978; 9:187–207.
3. Cunha CLP, Giuliani ER, Callahan JA, Pluth JR. Echophonocardiographic findings in patients with prosthetic heart valve malfunction. Mayo Clin Proc 1980; 55:231–242.
4. Cooper DM, Stewart WJ, Shiavone WA, et al. Evaluation of normal prosthetic valve function by Doppler echocardiography. Am Heart J 1987; 114:576–582.
5. Reisner SA, Meltzer RS. Normal values of prosthetic valve Doppler echocardiographic parameters: a review. J Am Soc Echocardiogr 1988; 1:203–210.
6. Ramirez ML, Wong M, Sadler N, Shah PM. Doppler evaluation of bioprosthetic and mechanical aortic valves: data from four models in 107 stable, ambulatory patients. Am Heart J 1988; 115:418–425.
7. Burstow DJ, Nishimura RA, Bailey KR, et al. Continuous wave Doppler echocardiographic measurement of prosthetic valve gradients: a simultaneous Doppler-catheter correlative study. Circulation 1989; 80:504–514.
8. Tatineni S, Barner HB, Pearson AC, et al. Rest and exercise evaluation of St. Jude Medical and Medtronic Hall prostheses: influence of primary lesion, valvular type, valvular size, and left ventricular function. Circulation 1989; 80(suppl I):16–23.
9. Sprecher DL, Adamick R, Adams D, Kisslo J. In vitro color flow, pulsed and continuous wave Doppler ultrasound masking of flow by prosthetic valves. J Am Coll Cardiol 1987; 9:1306–1310.
10. Nellessen U, Schnittger I, Appleton CP, et al. Transesophageal two-dimensional echocardiography and color Doppler flow velocity mapping in the evaluation of cardiac valve prostheses. Circulation 1988; 78:848–855.
11. Khandheria BK, Seward JB, Oh JK, et al: Value and limitations of transesophageal echocardiography in assessment of mitral valve prostheses. Circulation 1991; 83:1956–1968.
12. Taams MA, Gussenhoven EJ, Cahalan MK, et al. Transesophageal Doppler color flow imaging in the detection of native and Björk-Shiley mitral valve regurgitation. J Am Coll Cardiol 1989; 13:95–99.
13. Van den Brink RBA, Visser CA, Basart DCG, et al. Comparison of transthoracic and transesophageal color Doppler flow imaging in patients with mechanical prostheses in the mitral valve position. Am J Cardiol 1989; 63:1471–1474.
14. Daniel LB, Grigg LE, Weisel RD, Rakowski H. Comparison of transthoracic and transesophageal assessment of prosthetic valve dysfunction. Echocardiography 1990; 7:83–95.
15. Daniel WG, Nellessen U, Schroder E, et al. Left atrial spontaneous echo contrast in mitral valve disease: an indicator for an increased thromboembolic risk. J Am Coll Cardiol 1988; 11:1204–1211.
16. Daniel WG, Schröder E, Mügge A, et al. Transesophagel echocardiography in infective endocarditis. Am J Cardiac Imaging 1988; 2:78–85.
17. Lee E, Kee L, Schiller NB. Tranesophageal echocardiography and color flow imaging assessment of prosthetic and native valve dysfunction. Circulation 1988; 78(suppl II):607.

9 Aortic Dissection and Aneurysms

Acute dissection of the thoracic aorta represents a medical and surgical emergency requiring prompt diagnosis and treatment. In patients with untreated dissection of the aorta, mortality has been reported to be approximately 1 percent per hour during the first 48 hours, 80 percent within 2 weeks, and 90 percent within 3 months of clinical presentation,[1] warranting the rapid and accurate diagnosis of this condition.

Aortography and computed tomography (CT) have long been considered to be the standard diagnostic procedures in evaluating patients with thoracic aortic pathology, such as aortic dissection and aneurysms. The role of transthoracic echocardiography (TTE) in the diagnosis of aortic dissection is limited, owing to the inability of this procedure to visualize the thoracic aorta in its entirety. However, 2-D echocardiography does have a role in diagnosing and screening patients with suspected aortic dissection and has been found to be diagnostic if adequate images can be obtained.[2] Biplanar TEE has a distinct advantage over single-plane TEE in the examination of the entire thoracic aorta, including the ascending aorta, aortic arch, brachiocephalic vessels, and descending thoracic aorta, and, in some patients, the proximal abdominal aorta.

CLASSIFICATION SYSTEMS

Two anatomic classifications of aortic dissection that correlate with the prognosis and choice of therapy are currently used (Fig. 9-1). The DeBakey system includes three subtypes.[3]

In type I, the dissection begins in the ascending aorta, with propagation to the aortic arch, the descending thoracic aorta, and the abdominal aorta in most cases. In type II, the dissection is confined to the ascending aorta. In type III, the dissection begins at a point distal to the left subclavian artery. The Stanford University classification[4] is based on the presence or absence of involvement of the ascending aorta, accommodating subtypes with less frequent sites of intimal tears, yet preserving the important prognostic and therapeutic differences between involvement of the ascending aorta and of the descending aorta. In this classification, type A includes all the dissections that involve the ascending aorta with varying degrees of distal dissection, and type B includes all the dissections in which the ascending aorta is spared.

In a type A aortic dissection, the primary and/or entrant intimal tear is located in the ascending aorta in 84 percent, in the arch in 10 percent, and in the de-

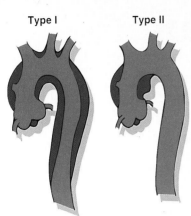

Type I   Type II

Type A- Ascending

Type III

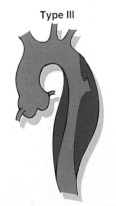

Type B- Descending

Fig. 9-1. Schematic diagram illustrating the Debakey *(top)* and Stanford *(bottom)* systems for classification of aortic dissection.

scending aorta beyond the origin of the left subclavian artery in 6 percent of cases. In a type B dissection, the primary and/or entrant tear is in the descending aorta beyond the origin of the left subclavian in 77 percent and in the arch in 23 percent of cases.[5]

VALUE AND LIMITATIONS OF TRANSTHORACIC ECHOCARDIOGRAPHY

Transthoracic echocardiography has been used extensively for detecting aortic lesions, using multiple transducer positions[6-8] (suprasternal, right and left parasternal, subcostal, infraclavicular, paraspinal, and abdominal). TTE and color Doppler imaging are useful techniques for evaluating complications of aortic dissection, including tamponade, aortic regurgitation, and status of left ventricular function. The presence of an intimal flap is highly predictive of dissection.[2,9-12] Color Doppler imaging permits assessment of the flow patterns within the true and false lumens and the severity of aortic regurgitation. It may identify the entrant and reentrant tears.[2] TTE can also demonstrate marked parallel widening of the aortic wall to more than 15 mm when the false lumen is completely thrombosed. However, other conditions can produce linear echo signals within the aortic lumen that can be mistaken for intimal flaps.[13] Scanning artifacts from the aortic valve or aortic root and fluid in the transverse pericardial sinus can also artifactually mimic dissection.[14] Although proximal aortic dissection can be diagnosed by TTE, this method is limited in visualizing the entire ascending aorta, aortic arch and descending thoracic aorta. TTE provides suboptimal image quality in patients with pulmonary emphysema, obesity, or thoracic deformity or in those on mechanical ventilation.

TRANSESOPHAGEAL ECHOCARDIOGRAPHY

TEE is highly sensitive and specific in the diagnosis of aortic dissection.[15-19] With the advent of biplane imaging, transverse and longitudinal sector scans of the aorta can be obtained. In most patients, direct imaging of most parts of the ascending aorta, transverse arch and arch vessels, and descending thoracic aorta can be clearly visualized and is markedly superior to the transthoracic approach. TEE should be performed whenever possible in patients with suspected acute aortic dissection before aortography, because acute aortic dissection is a medical emergency requiring prompt diagnosis and often immediate surgery. The procedure provides an optimal screening bedside test without the use of an intravenous contrast agent, an important factor because these patients may have compromised renal perfusion. We routinely administer sedation to avoid rapid shifts in blood pressure and heart rate. We have found TEE very useful at the bedside in the intensive care unit (ICU) and/or in the operating room, permitting immediate, accurate diagnosis of acute aortic dissection for emergency surgical intervention compared with aortic angiography and CT scanning, both of which may take several hours to organize and perform.

Transesophageal Aortic Anatomy

The normal transesophageal aortic scanning techniques and anatomy are discussed in Chapter 4 (see Fig. 4-32). The following points need to be emphasized when evaluating the aorta. The esophagus courses through the thorax from the pharynx to the stomach with slight side-to-side and anterior-to-posterior deviations. In the superior mediastinum, the esophagus is positioned between the vertebral column and the trachea, slightly to the left of the midline. The distal ascending aorta and proximal arch and innominate artery are directly in front of the air-filled trachea. In the mediastinum, the esophagus comes into virtual contact with the distal arch and isthmic portion of the descending aorta. It lies posterior and to the right of this segment of the arch. In the posterior mediastinum, the esophagus lies on the right side of the descending thoracic aorta. In the lower chest, it rests anteriorly and in front of the descending aorta, at the level of the diaphragm. Because of these changing relationships of the esophagus to aorta and the few internal anatomic landmarks, it is not possible to designate anteroposterior and right-to-left orientation of the descending thoracic aorta in TEE views. Thus, in practice, the distance from the transducer tip to the incisors is recorded throughout withdrawal to determine the site of observed aortic pathology.

Echocardiographic Findings

TEE can allow a prompt bedside diagnosis of dissection by demonstrating a mobile intimal flap separating the true and the false lumens[16-19] (Figs. 9-2 to 9-4). If the false lumen is completely thrombosed, central displacement of the intimal calcification is regarded as a positive finding. A side branch of the aorta can be assumed to be involved, if it is seen to contain a flap or if it arises from the false lumen. The proximal portion of the ascending aorta and the descending thoracic aorta are satisfactorily visualized

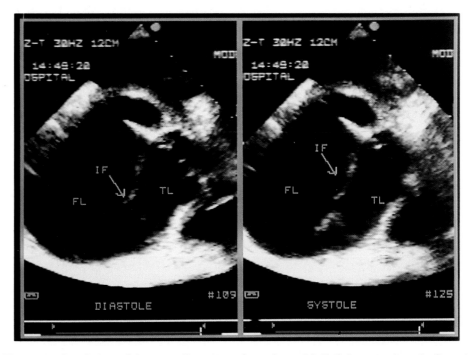

Fig. 9-2. Transverse basal view of the ascending aorta of a patient with DeBakey type I aortic dissection. *(Left)* The intimal flap (IF) separates the true lumen (TL) and false lumen (FL). Note the primary or entry tear. *(Right)* The IF moves toward the FL during systole.

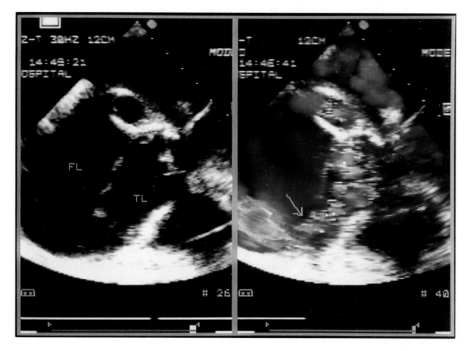

Fig. 9-3. DeBakey type I aortic dissection of same patient shown in Figure 9-2. *(Left)* Systolic freeze frame showing the primary tear and a large false lumen (FL). *(Right)* Color Doppler demonstrating flow across the intimal tear (arrow) into the FL. Note the sluggish or swirling type of flow pattern (dark blue) in the FL.

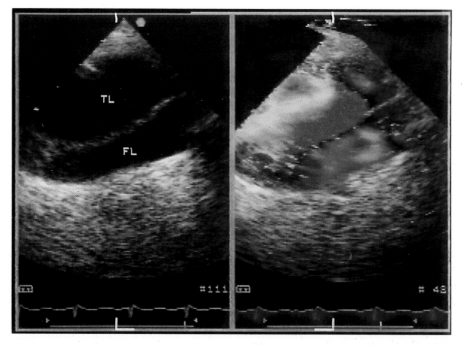

Fig. 9-4. Transverse view of the aortic arch in a patient with chest trauma. *(Left)* The true lumen (TL) is separated from the false lumen (FL) by the intimal flap. *(Right)* Color Doppler showing bidirectional flow during systole.

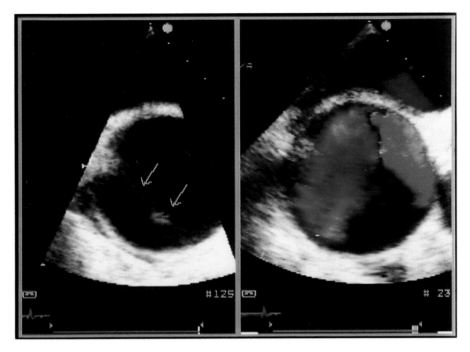

Fig. 9-5. Transverse view of ascending thoracic aorta. *(Left)* Side-lobing artifact (arrows) simulating an intimal flap. *(Right)* Color Doppler imaging demonstrating homogeneous color on both sides of this curvilinear echo without tears or entry points.

with a single-transverse plane probe; however, the distal portion of the ascending aorta and aortic arch are suboptimally imaged because of the interposition of the bronchus. This "blind" area in the distal ascending aorta is virtually eliminated with the use of the longitudinal plane. Occasionally, side lobing from the aortic valve can simulate an intimal flap in the ascending aorta, particularly with a transverse single plane probe with extreme anteflexion of the tip and high gain settings (Fig. 9-5). Side lobing is, however, a curvilinear echo along the sector arc, and it does not undulate like a true intimal flap. Color Doppler imaging also demonstrates homogeneous color on both sides of this curvilinear echo without any tears or communicating jets.

Complete TEE evaluation of the aorta using a biplane probe, pulsed Doppler, and color Doppler imaging can diagnose the presence, extent, and type of dissection in virtually every case. Furthermore, it provides information regarding the true and false lumen, entry or primary tear, and reentrant or secondary tears. TEE cannot provide information regarding in-volvement of the various thoracoabdominal aortic branches. True lumens can be differentiated from false lumens by the features summarized in Table 9-1.

Table 9-1. Features Differentiating True and False Lumens

The intimal flap moves toward the false lumen during systole, causing systolic expansion and diastolic compression of the true lumen.

The spontaneous echo contrast effect in the false lumen is caused by stasis and sluggish blood flow.

There is a variable degree of thrombus formation in the false lumen.

Color Doppler imaging frequently shows a slowly circulating or swirling type of flow pattern in the false lumen.

Color Doppler imaging shows biphasic flow across 75 percent of the secondary or reentrant tears, with a delayed systolic flow from true to false lumen, followed by reverse flow in diastole.

The false lumen is usually larger than the true lumen, especially in chronic cases.

(Adapted from Bansal and Shah,[23] with permission.)

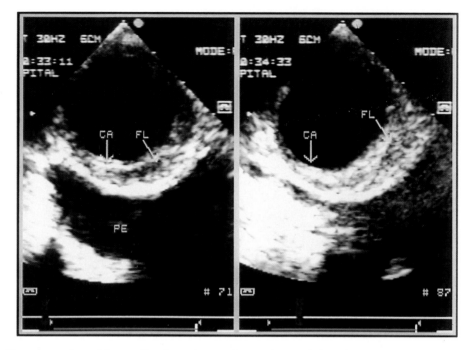

Fig. 9-6. Transverse view of descending thoracic aorta in a patient with DeBakey type III aortic dissection. The left image was recorded just distal to the origin of the left subclavian and the right image just proximal to the abdominal aorta. Note displacement of the intimal calcification (CA) and a thrombosed false lumen (FL). PE, pleural effusion.

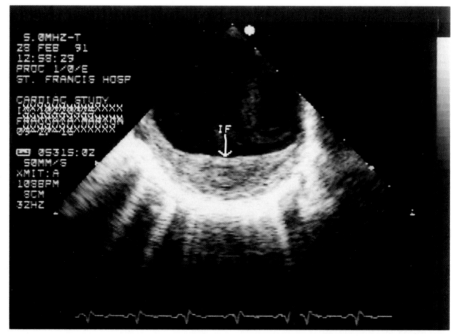

Fig. 9-7. Transverse view of descending thoracic aorta in a patient with DeBakey type III aortic dissection. The intimal flap (IF) separates the true lumen from a thrombosed false lumen. Note spontaneous echo contrast in the true lumen.

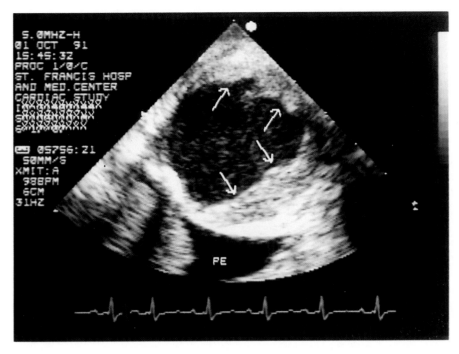

Fig. 9-8. Transverse plane of descending thoracic aorta demonstrating laminated thrombus (arrows) and spontaneous echo contrast (smoke) in patient with an aneurysm. PE, pleural effusion.

The differentiation of descending thoracic aortic aneurysm with a laminated clot from a completely thrombosed false lumen is possible by TEE. TEE permits cross-sectional images of the descending aorta at multiple levels; in patients with thrombosed false lumen, small, limited areas can be detected where a sluggish, swirling type of flow pattern by 2-D echo and low-velocity flows by color Doppler imaging provide clues that it is a false lumen rather than intraluminal clot. Also, displacement of the intimal calcification is consistent with a thrombosed false lumen (Figs. 9-6 and 9-7). All these features help in differentiating a thrombosed false lumen from an aneurysm filled with laminated thrombus (Fig. 9-8). The presence of a thrombus in an ascending aortic aneurysm is extremely unusual, and the appearance of thrombus should be regarded as strongly suspicious of a completely thrombosed false lumen of type A dissection (Fig. 9-9). We encountered one patient with a totally thrombosed false lumen in the ascending aorta that resulted in a false-negative diagnosis of dissection by angiography (Fig. 9-10).

Dissection flap interference with the aortic valve cusp motion and associated severe aortic regurgitation is also reliably assessed by TEE[19] (Figs. 9-11 and 9-12). The relationship of the dissection flap to the proximal left and right coronary arteries, the extension of dissection into the coronary arteries, or coronary blood flow obstruction produced by the dissection flap partially obstructing the coronary ostia are readily and reliably delineated and represent important clinical considerations in the treatment of these patients.

In our experience, this technique represents the current technique of choice in the assessment of patients with suspected acute thoracic aortic dissection. It has several advantages over aortography and CT scans: (1) the diagnosis can be promptly established at the bedside; (2) intimal flap, entry and reentry tears, and

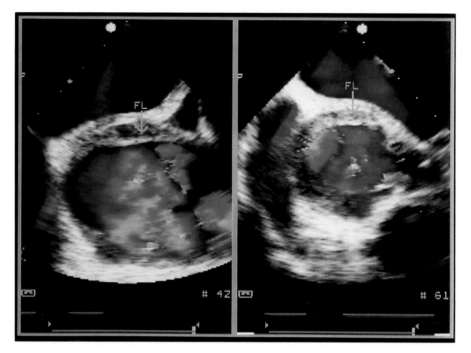

Fig. 9-9. Biplane imaging of DeBakey type I aortic dissection with thrombosed false lumen (FL). *(Left)* Longitudinal and *(right)* transverse imaging of ascending aorta. Color Doppler fills the true lumen without tears or entry points.

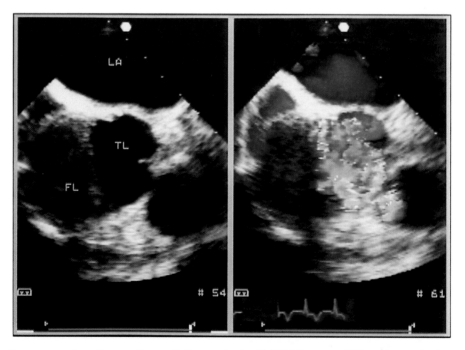

Fig. 9-10. Transverse view of ascending aorta in a patient with DeBakey type I dissection and a false-negative aortogram. *(Left)* Total thrombosis of the false lumen (FL). *(Right)* Color Doppler showing flow only in the true lumen (TL). LA, left atrium.

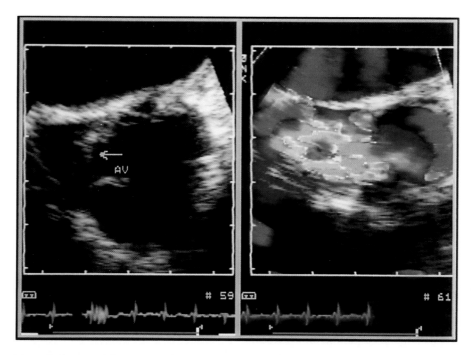

Fig. 9-11. Magnified view of the aortic valve (AV) using the longitudinal plane in patient with DeBakey type I aortic dissection. *(Left)* Diastolic frame demonstrating abnormal coaptation of the aortic valve cusp (arrow). *(Right)* Color Doppler image showing severe aortic regurgitation.

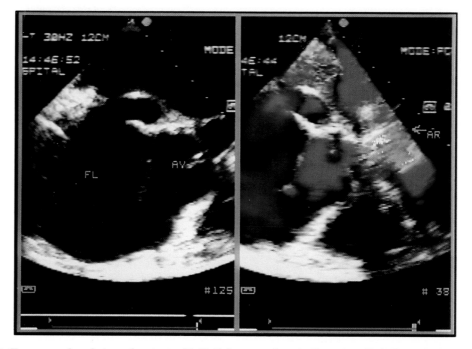

Fig. 9-12. Transverse basal view of patient with DeBakey type I aortic dissection. *(Left)* Diastolic frame showing a large false lumen (FL) and a small true lumen and aortic valve (AV). *(Right)* Color Doppler showing severe aortic regurgitation (AR).

flows can be defined; (3) aortic regurgitation can be detected and quantified; (4) left ventricular function can be assessed; (5) pericardial effusion and tamponade can be assessed; and (6) follow-up studies can be performed to assess the fate of the false lumen after medical and surgical intervention.

SERIAL FOLLOW-UP OF AORTIC DISSECTION

TEE also has an important role in the follow-up of patients with aortic dissection. Mohr-Kahaly et al.[18] followed up 18 patients with aortic dissection by serial TEE studies performed in the outpatient setting. The study showed the structure of the dissection, the surgical repair, and blood flow dynamics in the true and false lumen (Fig. 9-13). It showed the evolution of the dissection in many patients, 25 percent having complications of either extension of the dissection (5 percent), dilation of the aorta (11 percent), or aortic regurgitation (17 percent). In addition, in two patients, TEE documented healing of the dissection and obliteration of the false lumen with time. The absence of false lumen blood flow signals after surgery indicates successful closure of the true and false lumen communication, which may reduce the risk of dissection-rupture and thereby improve the patient's prognosis. This study shows the potential application of TEE to follow up these patients for disease progression, healing, or the need for surgical intervention.

DIAGNOSTIC ACCURACY

The diagnostic accuracy of TEE in aortic dissection has been evaluated in several studies. The European Cooperative Study Group[17] reported a multicenter study showing the diagnostic accuracy of single-plane imaging in 164 consecutive patients with suspected aortic dissection. The sensitivity and specificity were 99 percent and 98 percent, respectively, for TEE, compared with 83 percent and 100 percent, respectively, for CT scanning, and 88 percent and 94 percent, respectively, for aortic angiography.

Using aortography as the diagnostic goal standard, Hashimoto and co-workers[19] assessed the capability

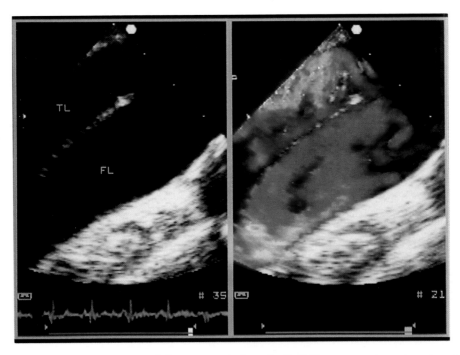

Fig. 9-13. Extension of aortic dissection following surgical repair. *(Left)* Transverse view of aortic arch showing the intimal flap separating the true lumen (TL) and false lumen (FL). Note a secondary reentry point. *(Right)* Color Doppler image showing bidirectional flow.

of biplane TEE in diagnosing dissection in 17 patients. With TEE, an intimal flap was recognized in all cases with aortic dissection and the entry site of acute dissection was identified in 14 of 17 cases.

TEE was used for 57 consecutive patients with acute aortic dissection.[15] These patients were examined with either the single-plane probe (39 patients) or the biplanar probe (18 patients) just after admission. The ascending and descending aortas were clearly visualized with either the single-plane or biplane probe, and all 57 patients with acute aortic dissection were identified. In 2 of 18 patients examined with the biplane probe, the entry was detected in the longitudinal view only. This study confirms the additional benefit of biplanar TEE in providing additional acoustic windows, ease of spatial orientation, and more accurate visualization of entry.

Biplane TEE appears to be the ideal initial screening test in a patient with suspected aortic dissection.[20] If type B dissection is diagnosed, the patient can be followed on medical management. If TEE demonstrates type A dissection, surgery can be performed, with or without angiography and CT.

AORTIC ANEURYSMS

Biplane TEE is useful in detecting aneurysms of the ascending and descending thoracic aorta (Figs. 9-14 and 9-15). The site of aneurysmal dilation and diameter of the aneurysm can be readily measured using the transverse and longitudinal planes (Fig. 9-16). In patients with an ectatic, tortuous, or aneurysmal aorta, the image planes may be oblique, making accurate cross-sectional measurement of luminal diameter difficult. Color Doppler imaging frequently demonstrates a slowly circulating or swirling type of flow pattern, and there is often spontaneous echo contrast in the dilated portion of the aorta (see Fig. 9-8).

The differentiation of descending thoracic aortic aneurysm with laminated clot from a completely thrombosed false lumen has already been discussed. Thrombus in an ascending aortic aneurysm is extremely unusual and should alert the clinician to the

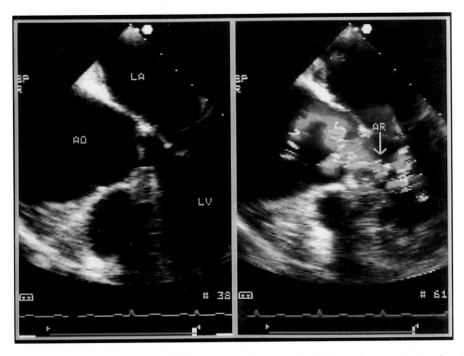

Fig. 9-14. Ascending aortic aneurysm. *(Left)* Transverse left ventricular (LV) outflow tract view showing aneurysmal dilation of the ascending aorta (AO). *(Right)* Color Doppler image demonstrating moderate aortic regurgitation (AR). LA, left atrium.

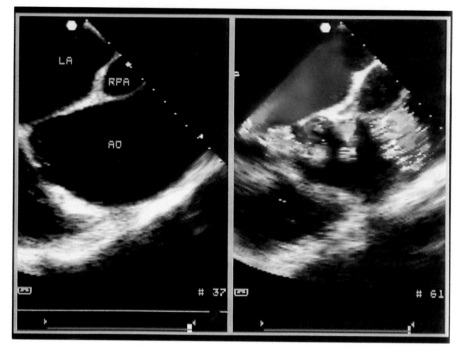

Fig. 9-15. Longitudinal view of the ascending aorta. *(Left)* Ascending aortic (AO) aneurysm measuring 6 cm in diameter. *(Right)* Color Doppler image revealing aortic regurgitation. LA, left atrium; RPA, right pulmonary artery.

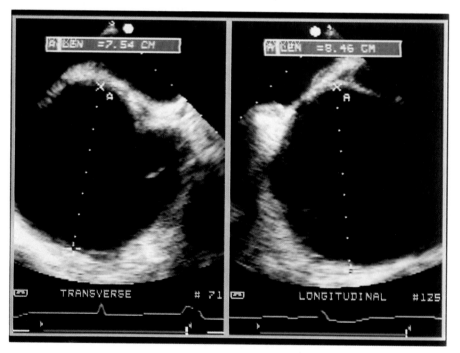

Fig. 9-16. Biplane imaging of ascending aortic aneurysm. The diameter of the aneurysm can be measured using the transverse and longitudinal planes (7.5 cm and 8.5 cm, respectively).

possibility of a completely thrombosed false lumen from type A dissection (see Figs. 9-9 and 9-10). TEE also permits visualization of aortic atheroma (see Ch. 12).

SAFETY OF TEE IN EVALUATING THORACIC AORTIC ANEURYSMS

Complications and adverse effects related to the use of TEE in patients with thoracic aortic aneurysms and dissection are infrequent even among very critically ill patients. Reported complications are discussed in Chapter 3. A case of rupture of an aortic dissection during a TEE procedure was reported by Silvey and associates.[21] During the TEE procedure, cardiac tamponade developed and, despite emergency pericardiocentesis, refractory tamponade persisted, resulting in death. Autopsy confirmed a type A dissection with a large posterior aortic tear communicating with the pericardium. Although spontaneous aneurysm rupture may have been unrelated to the TEE procedure, Silvey and colleagues postulate hemodynamic and mechanical effects of TEE that may have contributed to the aneurysm rupture. It is worth emphasizing that in patients with aortic dissection undergoing TEE, efforts should be made to minimize these hemodynamic and mechanical effects. These efforts should include adequate anesthesia and sedation to suppress the gag reflex and minimize gastric reaction; also, a minimal amount of torque on the TEE controls should be exerted. Urbanowicz et al.[22] noted that contact pressures between a TEE probe and the esophagus, although generally less than 17 mmHg, could reach 60 mmHg in individual patients. Such a high pressure exerted in the region of a large aortic aneurysm could have contributed to its rupture.

REFERENCES

1. Hirst AE, Johns VJ Jr, Kime SW Jr. Dissecting aneurysm of the aorta: a review of 505 cases. Medicine (Baltimore) 1958; 37:217–279.
2. Khandheria BK, Tajik AJ, Taylor CL, et al. Aortic dissection: review of value and limitations of two-dimensional echocardiography in a 6-year experience. J Am Soc Echocardiol 1989; 2:17–25.
3. DeBakey ME, Henly WS, Cooley DA, et al. Surgical management of dissecting aneurysms of the aorta. J Thorac Cardiovasc Surg 1965; 49:130–149.
4. Daily PO, Trueblood HW, Stinson EB, et al. Management of acute aortic dissections. Ann Thorac Surg 1970; 10:237–247.
5. Miller DC, Stinson EB, Oyer PE, et al. Operative treatment of aortic dissection. J Thorac Cardiovasc Surg 1979; 78:365–382.
6. Bansal RC, Tajik AJ, Seward JB, et al. Feasibility of detailed two-dimensional echocardiographic examination in adults. Mayo Clin Proc 1980; 55:291–308.
7. Come PC. Improved cross-sectional echocardiographic technique for visualization of the retrocardiac descending aorta in its long axis. Normal findings and abnormalities in saccular and/or dissecting aneurysms. Am J Cardiol 1983; 51:1029–1032.
8. Klein AL, Chan KL, Walley V. A new paraspinal window in the echocardiographic diagnosis of descending aortic dissection. Am Heart J 1987; 114:902–904.
9. Victor MF, Mintz GS, Kotler MN, et al. Two-dimensional echocardiographic diagnosis of aortic dissection. Am J Cardiol 1981; 48:1155–1159.
10. Mathew T, Nanda NC. Two-dimensional and Doppler echocardiographic evaluation of aortic aneurysm and dissection. Am J Cardiol 1984; 54:379–385.
11. Granato JE, Dee P, Gibson RS. Utility of two-dimensional echocardiography in suspected ascending aortic dissection. Am J Cardiol 1985; 56:123–129.
12. Iliceto S, Nanda NC, Rizzon P, et al. Color Doppler evaluation of aortic dissection. Circulation 1987; 75:748–755.
13. Bansal RC, Moloney PM, Marsa RJ, Jacobson JG. Echocardiographic features of a mycotic aneurysm of the left ventricular outflow tract caused by perforation of mitral-aortic intervalvular fibrosa. Circulation 1983; 67:930–934.
14. Wechsler RJ, Kotler MN, Steiner RM. Multimodality approach to thoracic aortic dissection. In Kotler MN, Steiner RM (eds): Cardiac Imaging: New Technologies and Clinical Application. Cardiovascular Clinics Vol. 17. Philadelphia: WB Saunders, 1986, pp 385–408.
15. Adachi H, Kyo S, Takamoto S, et al. Early diagnosis and surgical intervention of acute aortic dissection by transesophageal color flow mapping. Circulation 1990; 82(suppl IV):19–23.
16. Erbel R, Börner N, Steller D, et al. Detection of aortic dissection by transesophageal echocardiography. Br Heart J 1987; 58:45–51.
17. Erbel R, Engberdin R, Daniel W, et al, and the European Cooperative Study Group for Echocardiography: echocardiography in diagnosis of aortic dissection. Lancet 1989; 1:457–461.
18. Mohr-Kahaly S, Erbel R, Rennollet H, et al. Ambulatory follow-up of aortic dissection by transesophageal two-dimensional and color-coded Doppler echocardiography. Circulation 1989; 80:24–33.
19. Hashimoto S, Kumada T, Osakada G, et al. Assessment of transesophageal Doppler echography in dissecting aortic aneurysm. J Am Coll Cardiol 1989; 14:1253–1261.
20. Chandrasekaran K, Currie PJ. Transesophageal echocardiography in aortic dissection. J Invasive Cardiol 1989; 1:328–338.
21. Silvey SV, Stoughton TL, Pearl W, et al. Rupture of the outer partition of aortic dissection during transesophageal echocardiography. Am J Cardiol 1991; 68:286–287.
22. Urbanowicz JH, Kernoff RS, Oppenheim G, et al. Transesophageal echocardiography and its potential for esophageal damage. Anesthesiology 1990; 72:40–43.
23. Bansal RC, Shah PM. Transesophageal echocardiography. Curr Probl Cardiol 1990; 15:643–720.

10 Infective Endocarditis

Echocardiography supplements clinical and microbiologic data in the management of patients with endocarditis. Transthoracic echocardiography (TTE) is useful in patients with infective endocarditis to detect vegetations and assess the extent and hemodynamic sequelae of valvular damage. However, low diagnostic sensitivity has limited the value of echocardiography in patients in whom endocarditis is suspected but not certain.[1-3] Suboptimal patient imaging and limited instrument resolution are major obstacles to the application of TTE for this purpose. By contrast, TEE yields consistently high-quality images of the mitral, aortic, and tricuspid valves and is superior to TTE in the diagnosis of vegetations and abscesses from infective endocarditis.[4-10]

Endocardial vegetation is common to all types of infective endocarditis. The development of this characteristic lesion likely requires the simultaneous occurrence of several independent events.[11] First, the valve surface must be altered to produce a suitable site for bacterial attachment and colonization. This initial damage to the endothelial surface is probably provided by the actions of jet streams and eddy currents caused by various acquired and congenital valvular and other heart lesions. Intravenous (IV) drug users may traumatize the endothelial surface of valves through frequent injection of foreign particles. Such alterations result in the deposition of platelets and fibrin and in the formation of nonbacterial thrombotic endocarditis. Bacteria reach this site, adhere to the nonbacterial thrombus, and produce colonization. After colonization, the surface is rapidly covered with a protective sheath of platelets and fibrin to produce an environment conducive to further bacterial multiplication and growth of vegetation. Once the vegetation forms, valve destruction or distortion may occur; pieces may break off and give rise to emboli; bacteria may form abscesses or mycotic aneurysms at distant sites; and immune complexes may form, be deposited in vessels, and produce vasculitis. All these events result in the clinical manifestations of infective endocarditis.

NATIVE VALVE ENDOCARDITIS

In patients with suspected endocarditis, the detection of vegetations has important therapeutic and prognostic implications. Patients with vegetations tend to have a higher incidence of complications, including congestive heart failure, embolization, the need for surgical intervention, and death.[2,12-14] More recently, it has been reported that the prognostic implications are more dependent on vegetation size than on the presence or absence of vegetation alone.[5] Particularly for patients with mitral valve endocarditis, a vegetation diameter of greater than 10 mm was highly sensitive in identifying patients at risk of embolic events (Fig. 10-1). Vegetation size, however, was not significantly different in patients with and without severe heart failure or in patients surviving or dying during acute endocarditis. Robbins et al.[15] published their observations in 21 patients with a history of IV drug

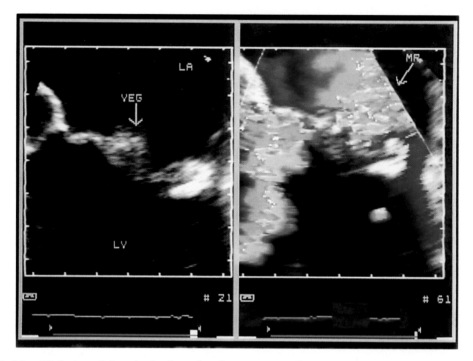

Fig. 10-1. Magnified view of the mitral valve using the transverse plane in a patient with *Streptococcus viridans* endocarditis. *(Left)* Large mitral valve vegetation (VEG) measuring greater than 10 mm. *(Right)* Color Doppler image showing an eccentric mitral regurgitant (MR) jet. LA, left atrium; LV, left ventricle.

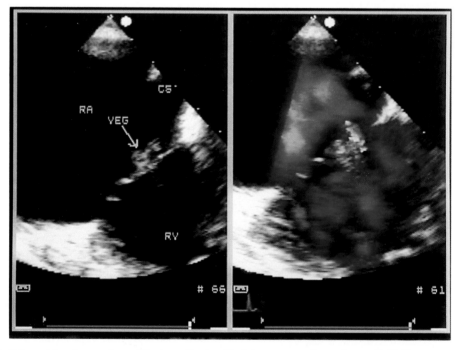

Fig. 10-2. Tricuspid valve endocarditis in patient with intravenous drug abuse. *(Left)* Transverse plane at coronary sinus (CS) level demonstrating a tricuspid valve vegetation (VEG). *(Right)* Color Doppler image revealing minimal tricuspid regurgitation. RA, right atrium; RV, right ventricle.

abuse and right-sided endocarditis affecting the tricuspid valve (Fig. 10-2). Four of the 11 patients (36 percent) with a tricuspid valve vegetation size of more than 10 mm required surgery because of persistent fever and bacteremia. No patient with an echocardiographically demonstrated vegetation size of less than 10 mm required surgery. Similarly, Stafford et al.[14] observed a higher incidence of embolic events and death only in patients with echocardiographically demonstrated vegetations of more than 5 mm in diameter. Because of these prognostic implications, precise detection and sizing of the vegetation have become important.

TEE is superior to TTE because of the better quality of resolution that can be obtained with TEE. TTE is extremely specific but insensitive in the diagnosis of infective endocarditis. TEE, on the other hand, has similar or greater specificity but is much more sensitive in detecting vegetations, particularly those that are small and those on prosthetic valves. The sensitivities for the two modalities are compared in Table 10-1.

TEE is able to detect 100 percent of vegetations greater than 11 mm in diameter, 69 percent of vegetations 6 to 10 mm in diameter, and 25 percent measuring 5 mm or less in diameter.[16] When echocardiographic findings are compared with surgical observation or necropsy findings, it has been shown that identification of vegetations by TEE is more reliable than identification by TTE (90 percent vs. 58 percent). These findings indicate the value of performing TEE in patients with suspected endocarditis. In view of the prognostic implications of detected vegetations, TEE should be performed on all patients with known or suspected infective endocarditis.

TEE is also superior in the detection and characterization of other rare complications of endocarditis (Figs. 10-3 to 10-5), including sinus of Valsalva aneurysm, mitral valve diverticulum and aneurysm, subaortic aneurysms arising from the mitral-aortic intervalvular fibrosa, and their rupture and communication with the left atrium.[17,18] Furthermore, multiple vegetations and valve perforations can be evaluated more clearly (Figs. 10-6 and 10-7).

Even with the use of high-resolution transducers, the diagnosis of a definite vegetation often is not possible without taking the patient's clinical presentation into account. In myxomatous valve disease, mitral valve thickening and prolapse cannot be reliably differentiated from vegetations without considering the clinical setting. It may also be impossible to differentiate old from new vegetations, vegetations from thrombi, or vegetations from valve disruption. In any individual patient, echocardiographic findings suggesting the presence of vegetation have to be carefully integrated with other clinical information.

Table 10-1. Comparison of Sensitivity of TTE and TEE for the Diagnosis of Infective Endocarditis

Reference	Year	No. of Patients	Sensitivity of TTE (%)	Sensitivity of TEE (%)
Daniel et al.[20]	1987	69	40	94
Erbel et al.[16]	1987–1988	96	44	82
Daniel et al.[19]	1988	76	60	94
Mügge et al.[5]	1989	80	58	90
Taams et al.[8]	1990	33	33	100
Shiveley et al.[4]	1991	62	44	94
Pedersen et al.[7]	1991	24	50	100

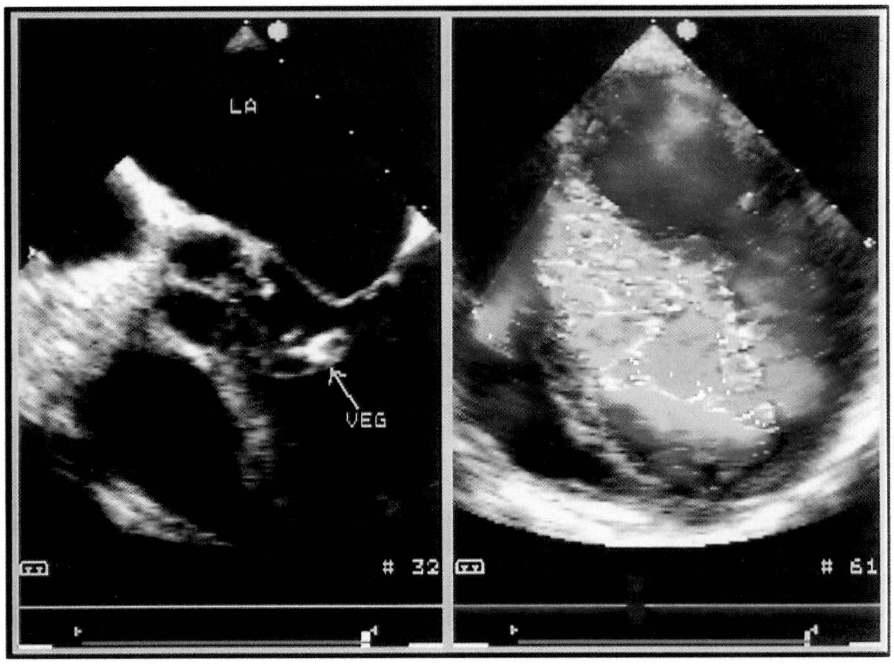

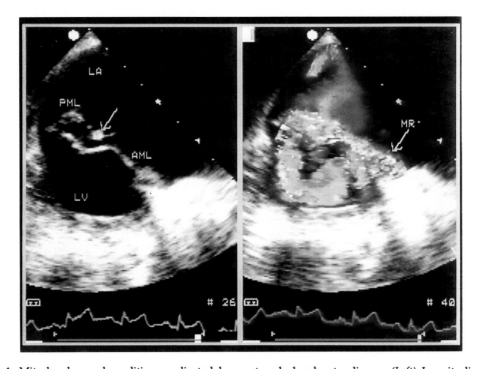

Fig. 10-3. Aortic valve endocarditis. *(Left)* Transverse five-chamber view showing a torn aortic leaflet and large vegetation (VEG) prolapsing in the left ventricular outflow tract during diastole. *(Right)* Color Doppler image demonstrating severe aortic regurgitation. The patient sustained a cerebral embolic event. LA, left atrium.

Fig. 10-4. Mitral valve endocarditis complicated by ruptured chordae tendineae. *(Left)* Longitudinal two-chamber view showing a flail posterior mitral leaflet (PML) and probably a small vegetation (arrow). *(Right)* Color Doppler image demonstrating severe eccentric mitral regurgitation (MR). AML, anterior mitral leaflet; LA, left atrium; LV, left ventricle.

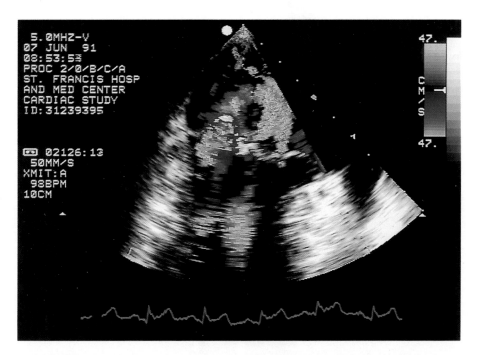

Fig. 10-5. Longitudinal two-chamber view showing mitral valve endocarditis with perforation of the anterior leaflet. Two mitral regurgitant jets are seen, one central and another through the body of the anterior leaflet.

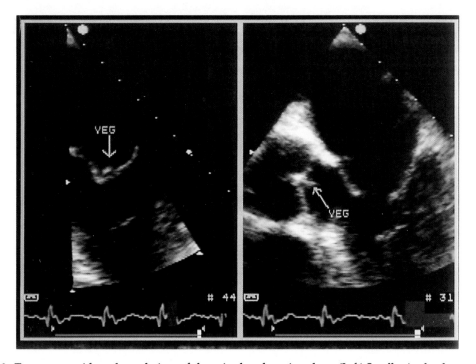

Fig. 10-6. Transverse midesophageal view of the mitral and aortic valves. *(Left)* Small mitral valve vegetation (VEG). *(Right)* Small vegetation (VEG) on the aortic valve. The vegetations were not noted on the transthoracic echocardiogram.

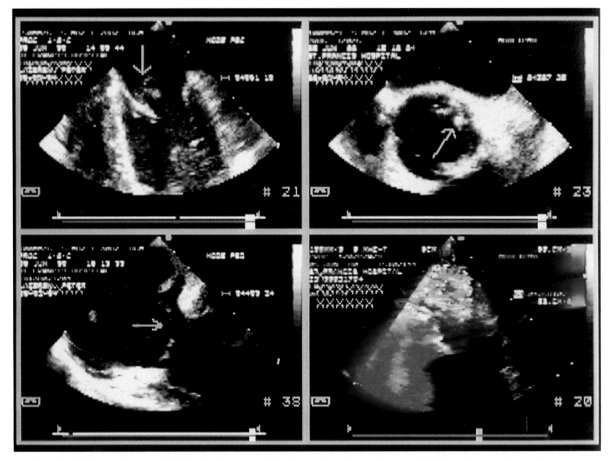

Fig. 10-7. Multivalvular endocarditis in an intravenous drug abuser. *(Upper left)* Transverse four-chamber view showing a vegetation on the anterior mitral leaflet (arrow). *(Upper right)* Basal view of the aortic valve demonstrating a small vegetation (arrow). *(Lower left)* Coronary sinus view showing a large tricuspid valve vegetation (arrow). *(Lower right)* Color Doppler image showing severe mitral regurgitation.

PROSTHETIC VALVE ENDOCARDITIS AND ABSCESSES

TEE has also been demonstrated to be of significant value in patients with prosthetic valve endocarditis and also for the detection of complications of endocarditis such as vegetations, ring abscesses, flail bioprosthetic cusps, sewing ring dehiscence, and periprosthetic leaks[6,7] (Figs. 10-8 and 10-9).

The characteristic echocardiographic findings of an abscess include a definite region of reduced echo density or echolucent cavities within the valvular annulus or adjacent myocardial structures in the setting of valvular infection (Figs. 10-10 and 10-11). These echocardiographic findings can be detected more often by TEE than by the transthoracic approach. Whereas the specificity and positive predicted value of the two techniques are similar, the sensitivity and negative predicted value of the transesophageal method are remarkably higher; sensitivity and specificity were 28 percent and 98 percent, respectively, for TTE and 87 percent and 94 percent for TEE.[6] Since patients with infective native or prosthetic valves usually have a worse prognosis when they have associated abscesses than when they do not, this feature of the transesophageal technique is of direct prognostic and therapeutic relevance. Patients with

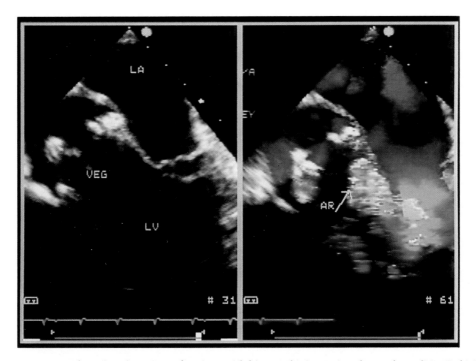

Fig. 10-8. Transverse five-chamber view of patient with bioprosthetic aortic valve endocarditis. *(Left)* A vegetation (VEG) shown prolapsing in the left ventricular (LV) outflow tract. *(Right)* Color flow image demonstrating moderate aortic regurgitation (AR). LA, left atrium.

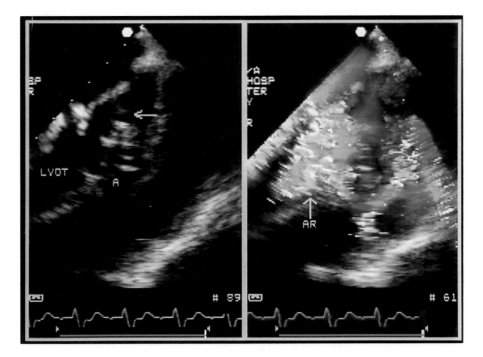

Fig. 10-9. *(Left)* Longitudinal plane of the left ventricular outflow tract (LVOT) and aorta in patient with dehiscence of a St. Jude aortic valve, vegetation (arrow), and aortic ring abscess (A). *(Right)* Color Doppler image showing severe aortic regurgitation (AR).

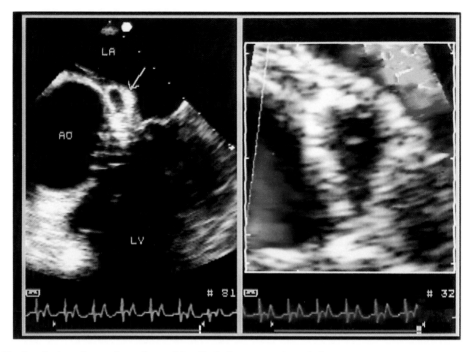

Fig. 10-10. Aortic ring abscess in patient with a St. Jude aortic valve. *(Left)* Cavity formation (arrow) around the aortic ring. The abscess is characterized by an echolucent cavity. *(Right)* Magnified view of abscess cavity without flow during color Doppler. AO, aorta; LA, left atrium; LV, left ventricle.

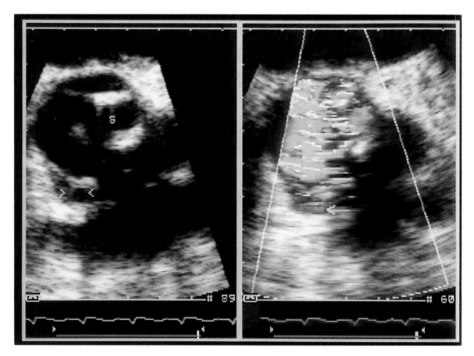

Fig. 10-11. Transverse basal short-axis view of a patient with bioprosthetic aortic valve endocarditis. *(Left)* All three struts (S) are identified. There is a small abscess cavity (arrowheads) on the anterior aortic ring. *(Right)* Color Doppler image in systole showing flow in the abscess cavity (arrow).

identified abscesses in the clinical setting of infective endocarditis are usually candidates for more aggressive therapy (including early surgery) than those without abscesses.

ECHOCARDIOGRAPHIC RECOMMENDATIONS

We believe that transthoracic 2-D echocardiography is useful as a routine screening test for patients with suspected infective endocarditis and that this procedure, when combined with Doppler and color Doppler imaging for detection and quantification of regurgitant lesions, is extremely useful in predicting prognosis. A negative transthoracic 2-D echocardiographic examination in a patient with strong clinical suspicion of infective endocarditis would warrant a TEE study; a normal TEE examination would make this diagnosis unlikely. The subgroup of patients who would particularly benefit from TEE include patients seen early in the course of disease who may have small vegetations and minimal valve destruction, as well those with poor transthoracic echocardiographic windows, patients on mechanical ventilators and patients with prosthetic valves. TEE is also indicated in patients with unreliable blood culture results (e.g., caused by recent antibiotic treatment) and in patients suspected of having ring abscesses.

REFERENCES

1. Come PC, Isaacs RE, Riley MF. Diagnostic accuracy of M-mode echocardiography in active endocarditis and prognostic implication of ultrasound-detectable vegetations. Am Heart J 1982; 103:839–847.
2. Stewart JA, Silimperi D, Harris P, et al. Echocardiographic documentation of vegetative lesions in infective endocarditis: clinical implications. Circulation 1980; 61:374–380.
3. Mintz GC, Kotler MN, Segal BL, Parry WR. Comparison of two-dimensional and M-mode echocardiography in the evaluation of patients with infective endocarditis. Am J Cardiol 1979; 43:738–744.
4. Shiveley BK, Gurule FT, Roldan CA, et al. Diagnostic valve of transesophageal compared with transthoracic echocardiography in infective endocarditis. J Am Coll Cardiol 1991; 18:391–397.
5. Mügge A, Daniel WG, Frank G, Lechtlen PR. Echocardiography in infective endocarditis: reassessment of prognostic implications of vegetation size determined by the transthoracic and the transesophageal approach. J Am Coll Cardiol 1989; 14:631–638.
6. Daniel WG, Mügge A, Martin RP, et al. Improvement in the diagnosis of abscesses associated with endocarditis by transesophageal echocardiography. N Engl J Med 1991; 324: 795–800.
7. Pedersen WR, Walker M, Olson JD, et al. Value of transesophageal echocardiography as an adjunct to transthoracic echocardiography in evaluation of native and prosthetic valve endocarditis. Chest 1991; 100:351–356.
8. Taams MA, Gussenhoven EJ, Bos E, et al. Enhanced morphological diagnosis in infective endocarditis by transesophageal echocardiography. Br Heart J 1990; 63:109–113.
9. Klodas E, Edwards WD, Khandheria BK. Use of transesophageal echocardiography for improving detection of valvular vegetation in subacute bacterial endocarditis. J Am Soc Echo Cardiogr 1989; 2:386–389.
10. Gussenhoven EJ, van Herwerden LA, Roelandt J, et al. Detailed analysis of aortic valve endocarditis: comparison of precordial, esophageal and epicardial two-dimensional echocardiography with surgical findings. J Clin Ultrasound 1986; 14:209–211.
11. Scheld WM, Sande MA. In Mandell GL (ed): Principles and Practice of Infectious Diseases. 2nd Ed. New York: Churchill Livingstone, 1985, p 504.
12. Brandenburg RO, Giuliani ER, Wilson WR, et al. Infective endocarditis: a 25 year overview of diagnosis and therapy. J Am Coll Cardiol 1983; 1:280–291.
13. Hickey AJ, Wolfers J, Wilcken DEL. Reliability and clinical relevance of detection of vegetations by echocardiography in bacterial endocarditis. Br Heart J 1981; 46:624–628.
14. Stafford WJ, Petch J, Radford DJ. Vegetations in infective endocarditis: clinical relevance and diagnosis by cross sectional echocardiography. Br Heart J 1985; 53:310–313.
15. Robbins MJ, Frater RWM, Soeiro R, et al. Influence of vegetation size on clinical outcome of right-sided infective endocarditis. Am J Med 1986; 80:165–171.
16. Erbel R, Rohmann S, Drexler M, et al. Improved diagnostic value of echocardiography in patients with infective endocarditis by transesophageal approach: a prospective study. Eur Heart J 1988; 9:43–53.
17. Teskey RJ, Chan KL, Beanlands DS. Diverticulum of the mitral valve complicating bacterial endocarditis: diagnosis by transesophageal echocardiography. Am Heart J 1989; 118:1063–1065.
18. Bansal RC, Graham BM, Jutzy KR, et al. Left ventricular outflow tract to left atrial communication secondary to rupture of mitral-aortic intervalvular fibrosa: diagnosis by transesophageal echocardiography. J Am Coll Cardiol 1990; 15:499–504.
19. Daniel WG, Schröder E, Mügge A, Lichtlen PR. Transesophageal echocardiography in infective endocarditis. Am J Cardiovasc Imaging 1988; 2:78–85.
20. Daniel WG, Schröder E, Nonnast-Daniel B, et al. Conventional and transesophageal echocardiography in the diagnosis of infective endocarditis. Eur Heart J 1987; 8(suppl):287–292.

11 Cardiac Tumors and Intracardiac Foreign Bodies

Since its introduction, echocardiography has been responsible for the initial detection of most intracardiac tumors.[1] TEE is superior to the transthoracic approach in reliably delineating the size, shape, point of attachment, and morphologic features of cardiac tumors.[2,3] These characteristics are best assessed by biplanar imaging. Examination of a mass in any single plane can provide equivocal findings or potentially misleading information, particularly if the mass is intersected obliquely or is eccentrically positioned.

Patients suspected of having a cardiac tumor should initially have a complete precordial examination. If there is a probable or definite mass identified by transthoracic echocardiography (TTE), but the clinical or echocardiographic features were atypical or not adequately explained, TEE can be requested for a better definition of attachment, location, intracardiac versus extracardiac, size and texture, as well as pertinent associations, such as tumor with thrombus.

BENIGN TUMORS

Myxomas

Myxomas comprise the single most commonly encountered tumor (Figs. 11-1 to 11-5). Seventy-five percent of the myxomas occur in the left atrium, 20 percent in the right atrium, and 5 percent elsewhere. Most atrial myxomas are attached to the atrial septum in the region of the fossa ovalis and are well detected by 2-D echocardiography.[4] Nonpedunculated myxomas (Fig. 11-6) as well as atypical locations, such as attachment to the eustachian valve, mitral valve, or biatrial extension, are better visualized with the transesophageal approach. In addition, TEE provides useful information in the intraoperative state in evaluating the integrity of the interatrial patch prior to the patient leaving the operating room (Figs. 11-7 and 11-8).

Papillomas

Papillomas are small frondlike ovoid tumors, usually attached to the valve leaflets or support apparatus. Although most papillomas are asymptomatic, their potential for coronary and cerebral embolization has been well documented.[5-7] In our experience, we have found papillomas to be more frequent on the mitral valve and to a lesser extent on the aortic and tricuspid valve leaflets. An ovoid frondlike mass in the absence of a recent infectious history is quite diagnostic of a benign papilloma.

Other Tumors

Other tumors with benign appearance and clinical presentation make up a diverse group of clinical and echocardiographic tumor types. These include fibroma, lipomatous hypertrophy of the atrial septum, and atrial septal lymphoma. Extracardiac masses can also be recognized and include solid tumors and pericardial cysts.

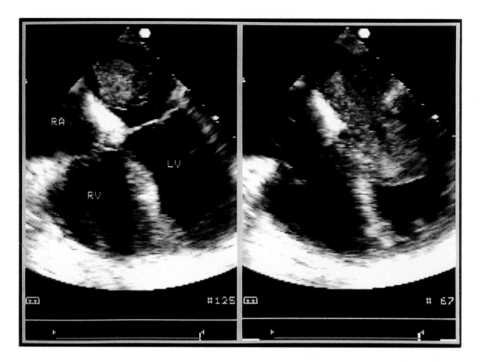

Fig. 11-1. Left atrial myxoma (T). *(Left)* Systolic frame, transverse four-chamber view of myxoma attached by stalk to interatrial septum. *(Right)* Diastolic frame of myxoma prolapsing into the left ventricle (LV). RA, right atrium; RV, right ventricle.

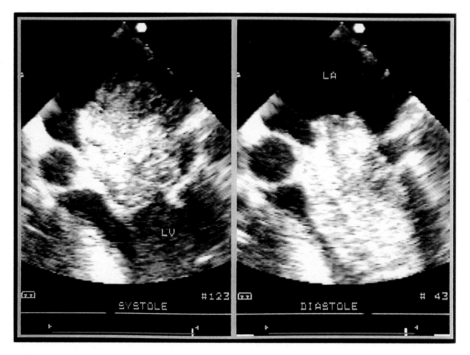

Fig. 11-2. *(Left)* Large left atrial myxoma occupying a large portion of the left atrium (LA) during systole. *(Right)* Prolapse into the left ventricle (LV) during diastole and obstructing left ventricular inflow.

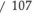

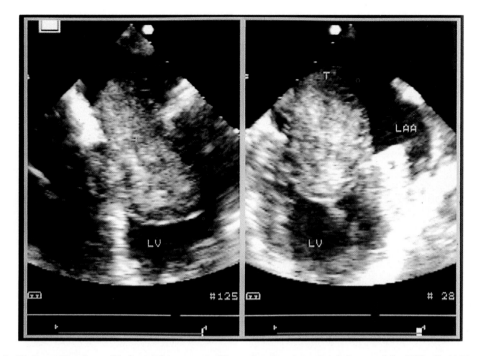

Fig. 11-3. Biplane imaging of left atrial myxoma (T) prolapsing into the left ventricle (LV). *(Left)* Transverse four-chamber view. *(Right)* Longitudinal two-chamber view. LAA, left atrial appendage; LV, left ventricle.

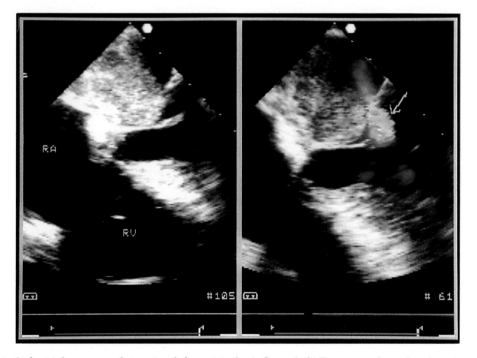

Fig. 11-4. Left atrial myxoma obstructing left ventricular inflow. *(Left)* Transverse four-chamber view demonstrating a large left atrial myxoma. *(Right)* Color Doppler image showing a narrow inflow jet across the mitral valve (arrow). RA, right atrium; RV, right ventricle.

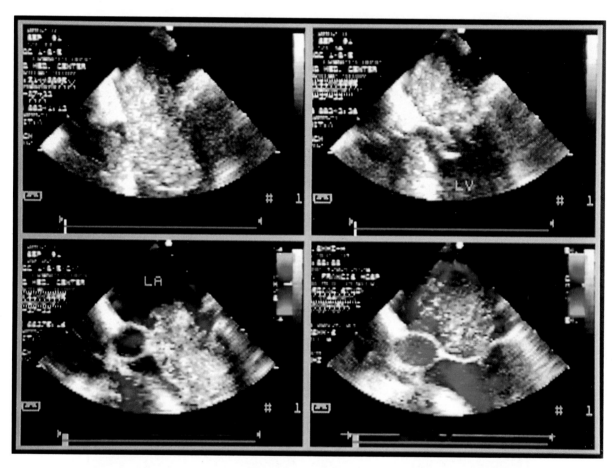

Fig. 11-5. *(Upper left)* Diastolic frame of pedunculated left atrial myxoma prolapsing into the left ventricle (LV). *(Upper right)* Systolic frame. *(Lower left)* Color Doppler image during diastole demonstrating reduced LV inflow caused by obstruction. *(Lower right)* Systolic frame showing minimal mitral regurgitation detected only at valve level. LA, left atrium.

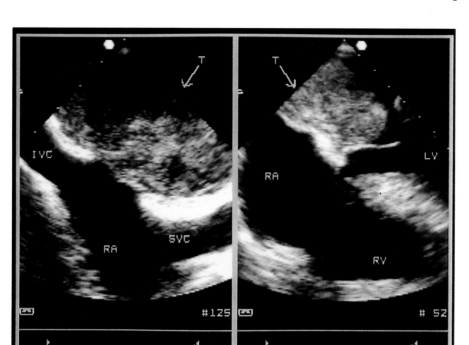

Fig. 11-6. Large nonpedunculated left atrial myxoma (T). *(Left)* Longitudinal basal view at level of superior vena cava (SVC) showing a broad base attachment of myxoma to interatrial septum. *(Right)* Transverse four-chamber view. IVC, inferior vena cava; LV, left ventricle; RA, right atrium; RV, right ventricle.

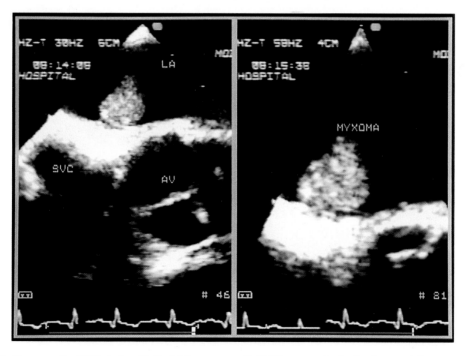

Fig. 11-7. Preoperative TEE study of left atrial myxoma. *(Left)* Myxoma attached to interatrial septum, taking on the appearance of a "Christmas tree." *(Right)* Magnified view of tumor. AV, aortic valve; LA, left atrium; SVC, superior vena cava.

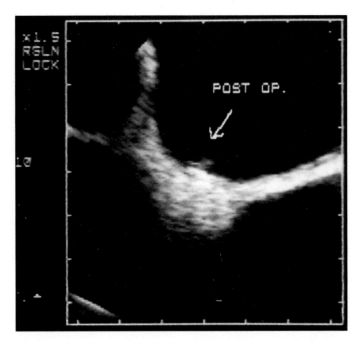

Fig. 11-8. Postoperative study, same patient as Figure 11-7. Removal of left atrial myxoma. There was no evidence of residual atrial septal defect on color Doppler (not shown).

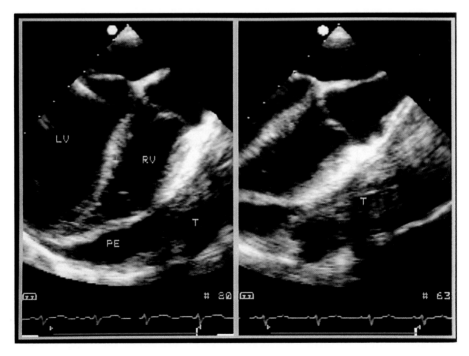

Fig. 11-9. Hodgkin's lymphoma (T) infiltrating the pericardial space and producing a pericardial effusion (PE). Note the extensive anterior mediastinal mass. LV, left ventricle; RV, right ventricle.

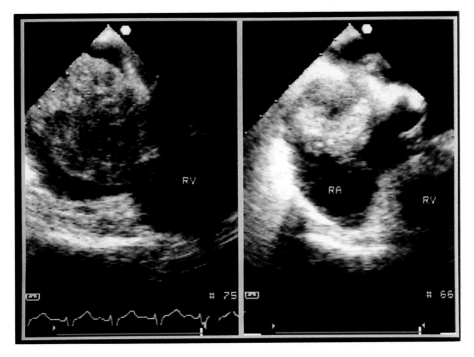

Fig. 11-10. Malignant thymoma involving the superior vena cava, right atrium (RA), and extending into the right ventricle (RV). *(Left)* Transverse four-chamber view. *(Right)* Transverse basal view.

MALIGNANT TUMORS

Although most malignant tumors originating from extracardiac structures and extending into cardiac chambers may be identified by either the transthoracic or the transesophageal approach, neither approach gives complete information about the precise extension of these tumors. For the evaluation of extracardiac metastatic tumors extending to the adjacent vascular and mediastinal structures, tomographic imaging modalities, such as computed tomography (CT) or magnetic resonance imaging (MRI),[8,9] are the supplemental diagnostic imaging methods of choice. The most common infiltrating tumor masses are from breast carcinoma, metastatic melanoma and lymphoma (Figs. 11-9 and 11-10).

Tumor compression of the heart can also be evaluated by biplane TEE. An anterior mediastinal mass can produce severe right ventricular and right ven-

tricular outflow tract compression. A posterior mediastinal mass usually compresses the posterior left atrial wall.

Malignant primary tumors comprise approximately 25 percent of all primary tumors of the heart and are chiefly sarcomas. The most common of these include angiosarcoma, rhabdomyosarcoma, and fibrosarcoma. These tumors are more common in adults and can involve either atrium or ventricle, but they are more common on the right side of the heart. Biplanar TEE is well suited for the diagnosis of right cardiac tumors.

INTRACARDIAC FOREIGN BODIES

TEE is useful in localizing the site of cardiac entrapment of fractured vascular catheters and other sources of embolization from various vascular de-

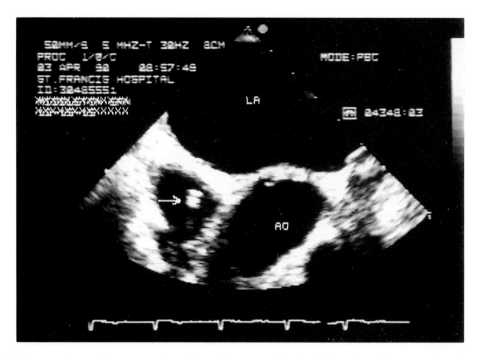

Fig. 11-11. Fractured central venous catheter (arrow) entrapped in the right atrium. Transverse basal view. AO, aorta; LA, left atrium.

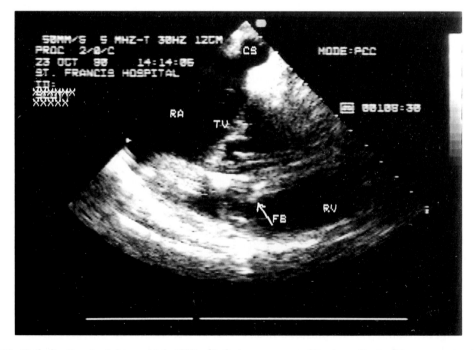

Fig. 11-12. Embolization to right ventricle (RV) of inferior vena cava filter in patient with recurrent pulmonary emboli. The foreign body (FB) is highly echogenic and entrapped across the tricuspid valve (TV). CS, coronary sinus; RA, right atrium.

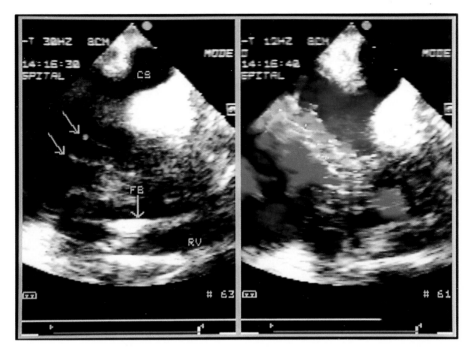

Fig. 11-13. Embolization to right ventricle (RV) of foreign body (FB), same patient as Figure 11-12. *(Left)* Traumatic rupture of chordae tendineae (arrows). *(Right)* Color Doppler image of severe tricuspid regurgitation. CS, coronary sinus.

vices. We have visualized fragments of venous catheters in the right atrium (Fig. 11-11) and embolization to the right ventricle of an inferior vena cava filter used in a patient with pulmonary emboli (Figs. 11-12 and 11-13).

Removal of a foreign body in the cardiac chambers requires precise localization, facilitated by biplane TEE. Removal of the foreign body can be accomplished via nonsurgical vascular retrieval or by surgical means.

REFERENCES

1. Nomeir AM, Watts LE, Seagle R, et al. Intracardiac myxomas: twenty-year echocardiographic experience with review of the literature. J Am Soc Echocardiogr 1989; 2:139–150.
2. Seward JB. Cardiac tumors, and thrombus: transesophageal echocardiographic experience. In Erbel R, Khandheria BK, Brennecke R (eds): Transesophageal Echocardiography: A New Window to the Heart. New York: Springer-Verlag, 1989, pp 120–128.
3. Obeid A, Marvasti M, Parker F, et al. Comparison of transthoracic and transesophageal echocardiography in diagnosis of left atrial myxoma. Am J Cardiol 1989; 63:1006–1008.
4. Fyke FE III, Seward JB, Edwards WD, et al. Primary cardiac tumors: experience with 30 consecutive patients since the introduction of two-dimensional echocardiography. J Am Coll Cardiol 1985; 5:1465–1473.
5. McFadden PM, Lacy JR. Intracardiac papillary fibroelastoma: an occult cause of embolic neurologic deficit. Ann Thorac Surg 1987; 43:667–669.
6. Kasarskis EJ, O'Connor W, Earle G. Embolic stroke from cardiac papillary fibroelastomas. Stroke 1988; 19:1171–1173.
7. Mazzucco A, Faggian G, Bortolotti U, et al. Embolizing papillary fibroelastoma of the mitral valve. Tex Heart Inst J 1991; 18: 62–66.
8. Freedberg RS, Kronzon I, Rumancik WM, Liebeskind D. The contribution of magnetic resonance imaging to the evaluation of intracardiac tumors diagnosed by echocardiography. Circulation 1988; 77:96–103.
9. Winkler M, Higgins CB. Suspected intracardiac masses: evaluation with MR imaging. Radiology 1987; 165:117–122.

12 Evaluating the Source of Embolization

Echocardiographic examinations are frequently obtained in patients with unexplained arterial embolism and embolic stroke. Transthoracic echocardiography (TTE) is frequently used to evaluate patients with suspected embolic events originating in the heart. The yield of TTE has been limited, however, owing to a variety of reasons, including inability to visualize the left atrial appendage, suboptimal images in patients with chest deformities, chronic obstructive pulmonary disease, obesity, and attenuation and masking from prosthetic material. The importance of a cardiac source of embolism has been emphasized by the second report of the Cerebral Embolism Task Force, which has found that as many as one in six patients with cerebral embolism have a cardiac etiology for their symptoms.[1]

TEE has developed as a means of evaluating patients with unexplained emboli, for which it has proven superior to the TTE approach.[2] As a result, more and more patients are being referred for TEE for determination of a source of embolization, which was the indication for the procedure in 35 percent of patients from our laboratory. This Chapter will focus on the major intracardiac sources of emboli that can be accurately diagnosed with TEE, as well as a newly recognized extracardiac source of cerebral and peripheral emboli that has been discovered only through the advent of TEE: protruding atheromas in the thoracic aorta (Table 12-1).

DETECTION OF LEFT ATRIAL THROMBUS

Left atrial thrombi have been shown to occur in the setting of atrial dilation that accompanies rheumatic valvular disease, atrial fibrillation, and cardiomyopathy.[3] Left atrial thrombi have been reported to be present in 10 percent to 25 percent of patients with rheumatic mitral valve disease, as shown by clinicopathologic studies.[4] A high percentage of these patients, approximately 50 percent, is subject to systemic arterial embolism.[5] Therefore, the detection of left atrial thrombi is important, especially when surgical mitral commissurotomy or mitral balloon valvuloplasty is being considered. Furthermore, in patients considered for electrical cardioversion of atrial flutter/fibrillation and in whom left atrial or appendage thrombi are identified, a 2- to 3-week course of anticoagulation before attempted cardioversion is a logical approach to minimizing the risk of arterial embolization.

Table 12-1. Sources of Embolization Diagnosed by TEE

Left atrial thrombus, left atrial appendage thrombus
Left atrial spontaneous echo contrast
Patent foramen ovale
Atrial septal aneurysm
Mitral valve prolapse
Vegetation
Prosthetic valve thrombus
Left ventricular apical thrombi
Protruding atherosclerotic plaque in the thoracic aorta

The limitations of TTE may be explained by a relatively low resolution in the far field of the transducer and by the fact that the left atrial appendage is difficult to visualize in adult patients.[6] Visualization of the left atrial appendage is important because approximately 50 percent of left atrial thrombi in patients with stenotic mitral valve disease and a history of embolization are limited to this structure.

By contrast, TEE has overcome these limitations and is a highly sensitive technique in identifying left atrial thrombi.[6] This advantage may be explained by the close proximity of the esophagus to the left atrium which allows highly detailed visualization of the left atrium and its appendage. As a consequence, TEE has evolved as the procedure of first choice for the noninvasive diagnosis of left atrial thrombi. In addition to identifying the presence of atrial thrombi, TEE permits reliable evaluation of the extent, site of attachment, and mobility of atrial thrombi (Figs. 12-1 to 12-6).

The left atrial appendage is a highly contractile pump with a pattern of contraction quite distinct from that of the main body of the left atrium.[7] Left atrial appendage thrombus formation is associated with decreased left atrial appendage contraction as well as with left atrial appendage dilatation (Fig. 12-7). A severely hypokinetic left atrial appendage, usually also associated with an enlarged left atrial appendage, would predispose to thrombus formation just as left ventricular aneurysm predisposes to thrombus formation.

TEE also permits visualization of the upper left atrial wall near the entrance of the upper pulmonary veins, an area that is not visualized during TTE examinations, and is another site for thrombus formation.

TEE is a valuable technique for detecting left atrial thrombi in candidates for percutaneous balloon mitral valvuloplasty. In one study,[8] thrombi were found in 5 of 19 candidates for this procedure (26 percent);

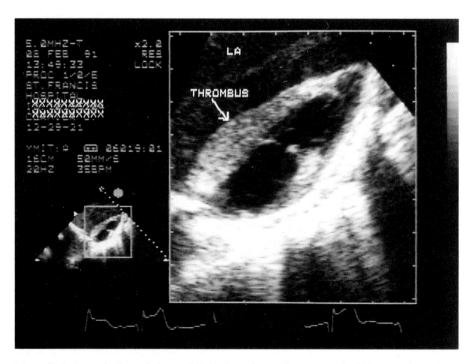

Fig. 12-1. Magnified view of a large left atrial (LA) thrombus. There is marked degree of swirling, indicating stasis.

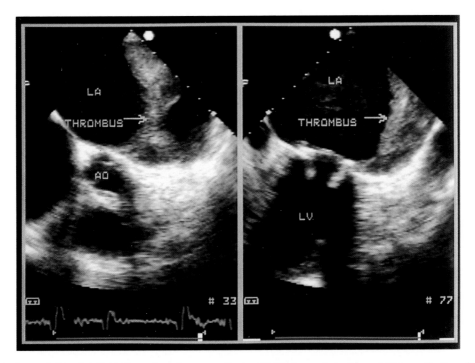

Fig. 12-2. Large left atrial (LA) thrombus from a patient with history of stroke and bioprosthetic valve. *(Left)* Transverse basal short-axis view revealing a large thrombus. *(Right)* Four-chamber view showing the large laminated thrombus. Note the struts of the bioprosthetic valve. AO, aorta; LV, left ventricle.

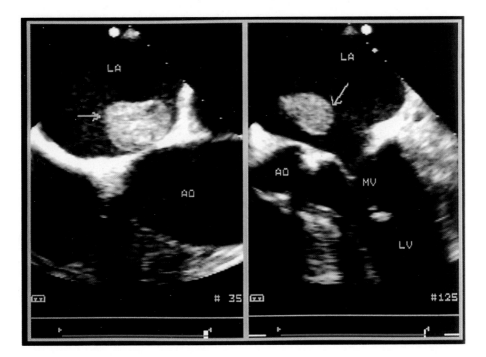

Fig. 12-3. Large left atrial (LA) thrombus (arrow) simulating left atrial myxoma. *(Left)* Longitudinal basal view. *(Right)* Transverse five-chamber view. The thrombus is mobile and there is spontaneous echo contrast. AO, aorta; LV, left ventricle; MV, mitral valve.

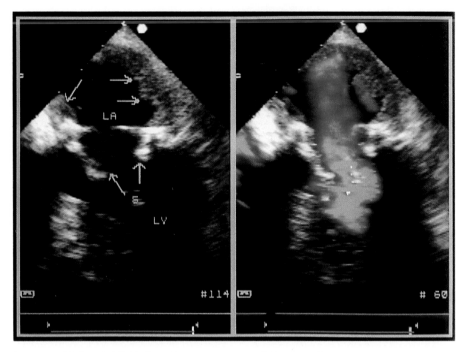

Fig. 12-4. Laminated left atrial (LA) thrombus in patient with history of stroke and Carpentier-Edwards prosthetic valve. *(Left)* Transverse midesophageal view demonstrating thrombus (arrows) within left atrial cavity and struts (S) of bioprosthetic valve. *(Right)* Color Doppler image during diastole. LV, left ventricle.

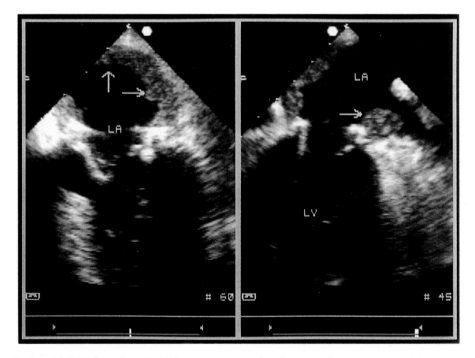

Fig. 12-5. Left atrial (LA) thrombus. *(Left)* Transverse four-chamber view from patient with bioprosthetic valve and atrial fibrillation showing a large laminated thrombus (arrows). *(Right)* Longitudinal two-chamber view demonstrating thrombus (arrow) in the left atrial appendage. LV, left ventricle.

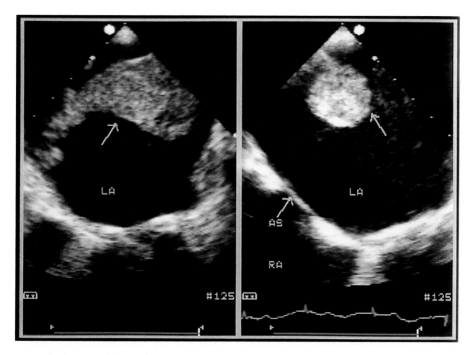

Fig. 12-6. Magnified view of the left atrium (LA) from a transverse four-chamber view from a patient with rheumatic mitral valve disease showing an extensive thrombus (arrow). AS, atrial septum.

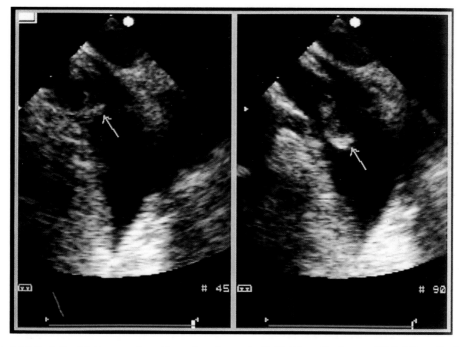

Fig. 12-7. Mobile left atrial appendage thrombus (arrow). *(Left)* Diastolic frame. *(Right)* Systolic frame. The appendage is dilated.

in only one of these five patients was there suspicion of left atrial thrombus on TTE. There was a thrombus in the appendage in all five patients, and it was limited to the appendage in three. Balloon valvuloplasty was not performed in four of the five patients with clot seen on TEE because of the potential for embolization, as it has been shown by TEE during balloon mitral valvuloplasty that the guide wires may enter the atrial appendage during the various manipulations that occur during the procedure.[9] Embolization has been reported in 4.2 percent of patients undergoing balloon valvuloplasty.[10]

In summary, because up to 50 percent of all left atrial thrombi are limited to the appendage, and because the appendage is difficult to visualize by standard TTE, TEE is the procedure of choice for the diagnosis of left atrial clot in patients who have emboli or who are at risk of having one. Furthermore, as the superior aspect of the atrium is also not visualized by the transthoracic approach and is clearly seen from the esophagus, TEE is well suited for the detection of clots hiding in this area.

LEFT ATRIAL SPONTANEOUS ECHO CONTRAST

Dynamic smokelike echoes in the left atrial cavity, known as spontaneous echo contrast, are an occasional finding during TTE.[11-13] TEE provides superior imaging of the left atrium, and left atrial spontaneous echo contrast has been detected more frequently by this technique.[14-18] Left atrial spontaneous echo contrast has been noted in patients with rheumatic heart disease, prosthetic valves, atrial fibrillation, or low cardiac output (Figs. 12-8 and 12-9). This phenomenon is believed to result from sludging of red cells[15] or circulating platelet and platelet-neutrophil aggregates[19] and has been shown to be associated with an increased risk of arterial embolization.[15,20]

Daniel and co-workers[15] evaluated the incidence of spontaneous echo contrast in the left atrium in 122 patients with mitral stenosis or after mitral valve replacement using TEE. They reported that patients with spontaneous echo contrast had a significantly greater incidence of both left atrial thrombi and a

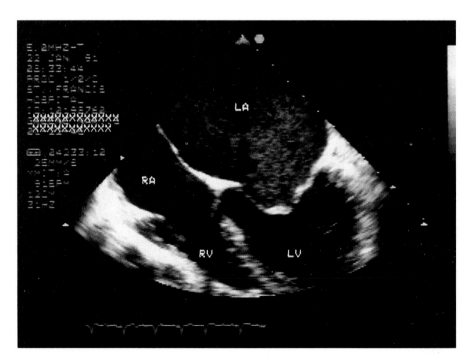

Fig. 12-8. Transverse four-chamber view from a patient with rheumatic mitral stenosis and a history of stroke. There is marked degree of spontaneous echo contrast in the left atrium (LA). LV, left ventricle; RA, right atrium; RV, right ventricle.

history of arterial embolic episodes than did patients without spontaneous echo contrast. Therefore, spontaneous echo contrast in the left atrium detected by TEE might be useful in identifying increased thromboembolic risk. However, Daniel et al.[15] also reported that there were embolic episodes in four patients with mitral stenosis who did not have spontaneous echo contrast; therefore, the probability is that we cannot use the nondetection of spontaneous echo contrast in the left atrium to make a determination to not anticoagulate.

Matsuzaki and associates[21-23] reported the relation between blood velocity in the left atrial appendage and thromboembolic risk in 28 patients with chronic atrial fibrillation. In patients with lone atrial fibrillation and a history of cerebral thromboembolism, a small mural thrombus in the left atrial appendage was observed in 22 percent, and only one patient had spontaneous echo contrast in the left atrium. However, mean flow velocity (averaged flow of a sawtooth velocity pattern) in the left atrial appendage was significantly lower in the patient with lone atrial

fibrillation and a history of thromboembolic episodes (11 ± 4 cm/s) than that in patients with lone atrial fibrillation and no history of thromboembolic episodes (29 ± 9 cm/s), indicating severe blood stagnation in the appendage in the group with a history of thromboembolism. Thus, measurements of the flow velocity signal in the left atrial appendage with TEE may be useful in identifying increased thromboembolic risk in patients with atrial fibrillation.

PATENT FORAMEN OVALE

At necropsy, a patent foramen ovale is found in about 30 percent of cases.[24] Since physical examination in patients with patent foramen ovale reveals no abnormal findings, its diagnosis during life is usually restricted to cardiac catheterization. Occasionally, patent foramen ovale can also be visualized by contrast echocardiography where a small right-to-left atrial shunt of the microbubbles may be identified during the Valsalva maneuver.[25,26] The Valsalva maneuver, however, is frequently associated with a marked impairment of the imaging quality in TTE preventing a

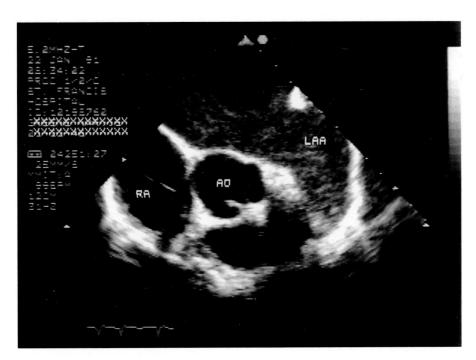

Fig. 12-9. Transverse basal short-axis view at the level of the left atrial appendage (LAA) showing spontaneous echo contrast. AO, aorta; RA, right atrium.

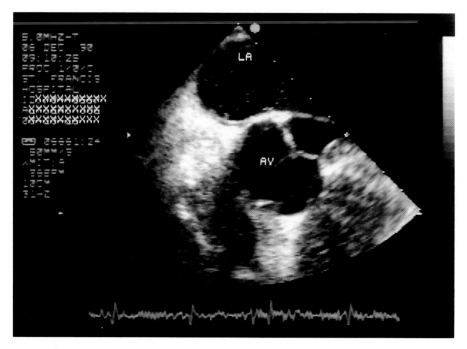

Fig. 12-10. Transverse basal short-axis view using agitated saline contrast through an antecubital vein opacifying the right atrium and passage of saline contrast microbubbles across a patent foramen ovale into the left atrium (LA). AV, aortic valve.

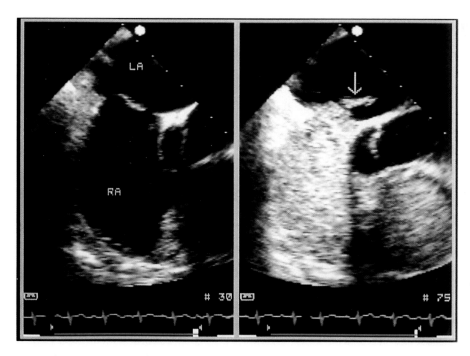

Fig. 12-11. Patent foramen ovale. *(Left)* Transverse basal short-axis view prior to contrast administration. *(Right)* Agitated saline contrast demonstrating passage of microbubbles across a patent foramen ovale (arrow) after Valsalva release, resulting in right-to-left shunting. RA, right atrium.

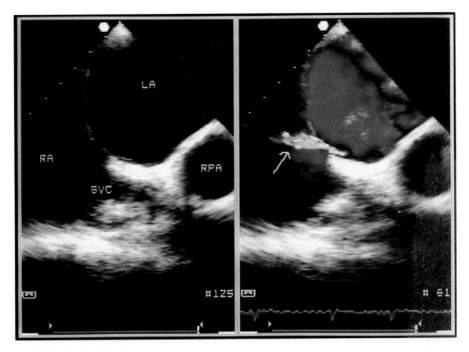

Fig. 12-12. *(Left)* Longitudinal basal view at level of superior vena cava (SVC) and atrial septum. *(Right)* Color Doppler image demonstrating a patent foramen ovale (arrow). LA, left atrium; RA, right atrium; RPA, right pulmonary artery.

definite diagnosis. Although in most patients a patent foramen ovale remains without clinical relevance, it may be the window for paradoxical emboli. Thus, at least in patients with unexplained arterial embolism, the detection of patent foramen ovale seems helpful in establishing the correct diagnosis.

TEE with contrast appears to be more sensitive for the detection of patent foramen ovale[27] (Figs. 12-10 and 12-11). A group from the Mayo Clinic reported an incidence of 28 percent in 606 patients studied.[28] Furthermore, the prevalence of patent foramen in patients referred for the source of the embolism was not significantly different from that in patients referred for other indications: 27 percent versus 29 percent. The echocardiographic prevalence of patent foramen ovale is comparable to the 30 percent found at autopsy.[24]

Three distinct mechanisms of right-to-left interatrial shunting in the absence of right ventricular systolic hypertension have been identified[29]: (1) transient spontaneous reversal of the left-to-right atrial pressure differential with each cardiac cycle, (2) sustained elevation of right atrial pressure above left atrial pressure induced by respiratory maneuvers, and (3) aberrant flow redirection across the foramen ovale caused by a large right atrial mass. Any of these three mechanisms may be operative during paradoxic embolism in the absence of elevation of right ventricular pressures.

The longitudinal plane is the preferred scanning orientation for visualization of patency of the foramen ovale (Figs. 12-12 and 12-13). Venous contrast echocardiography with Valsalva release best detects right-to-left shunting.

If patent foramen ovale proves to be the only abnormality on TEE, further work up such as search for lower extremity venous thrombosis or pulmonary

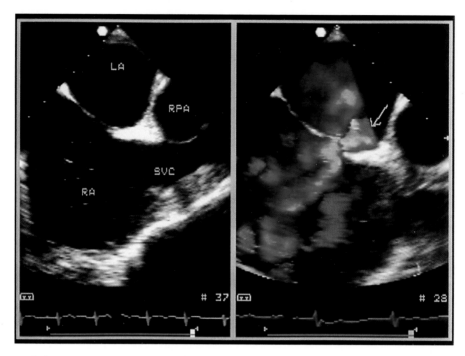

Fig. 12-13. *(Left)* Longitudinal view at level of superior vena cava (SVC) and atrial septum. *(Right)* Color Doppler map demonstrating a patent foramen ovale (arrow). LA, left atrium; RA, right atrium; RPA, right pulmonary artery.

embolization, is indicated to establish the diagnosis of paradoxical embolization.

ATRIAL SEPTAL ANEURYSM

Aneurysm involving the fossa ovalis was first reported in 1934.[30] Autopsy findings have noted that the surfaces of the aneurysm were often roughened by tiny fibrin-thrombus tags, and a gross thrombus was noted at the base of one aneurysm.[31] In addition, 50 percent had a patent foramen ovale.

Atrial septal aneurysms are associated with an increased incidence of atrial septal defect,[32] atrioventricular valve prolapse,[33] atrial tachyarrhythmias,[33,34] atrial thrombus formation, and subsequent systemic and cerebrovascular embolic events.[35,36] The association of mitral valve prolapse and atrial septal aneurysm appears to be particularly important in that this subset of patients have an increased likelihood of cerebrovascular embolic events.[37] One characteristic of the aneurysm, the thickness of the aneurysmal membrane, was significantly associated with emboli.[37] The thickness was 5 mm or more in 9 of 12 patients with emboli (75 percent) and in only 3 of 11 without emboli (27 percent).

TEE has played an important role in the diagnosis of atrial septal aneurysm (Figs. 12-14 and 12-15) and in helping define its embolic potential.[38,39] In one series of 199 studies,[38] an atrial septal aneurysm was seen in 20 patients (10 percent), only 1 percent of the 2,059 transthoracic echocardiograms performed in the same laboratory. Documented ischemic brain events developed in 5 of the 20 patients (25 percent); all 5 had shunting from right-to-left on contrast injection. Atrial septal aneurysms may bulge into the left and/ or right atria, and its motion is probably secondary to changes in transatrial pressure gradients with the cardiac cycle.[35,36]

Atrial septal aneurysms can be mistaken for atrial cysts or tumor masses,[35,39] and TEE is currently the most accurate method of identifying this entity.

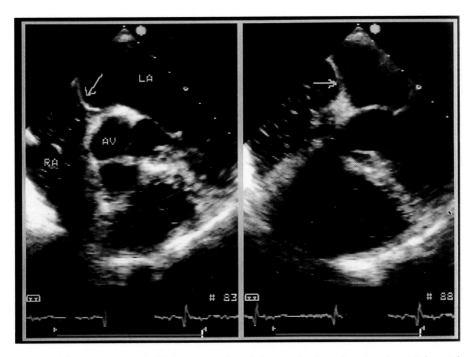

Fig. 12-14. Atrial septal aneurysm. *(Left)* Transverse basal short-axis view showing the atrial septal aneurysm (arrow) bulging into the right atrium (RA) during systole. *(Right)* Transverse four-chamber view demonstrating the aneurysm (arrow) bulging into the left atrium (LA) during diastole. Note spontaneous echo contrast in the right atrium. AV, aortic valve.

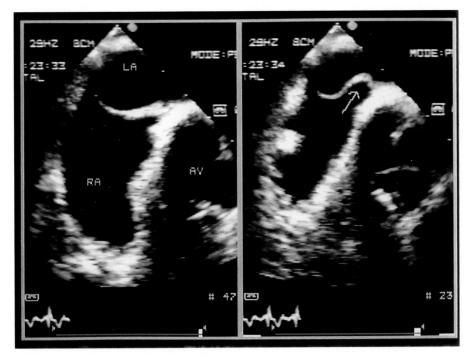

Fig. 12-15. Transverse basal short-axis view demonstrating an atrial septal aneurysm. *(Left)* Systolic frame showing the atrial septum bulging into the right atrium (RA). *(Right)* Diastole frame demonstrates the aneurysm (arrow) bulging into the left atrium (LA). AV, aortic valve.

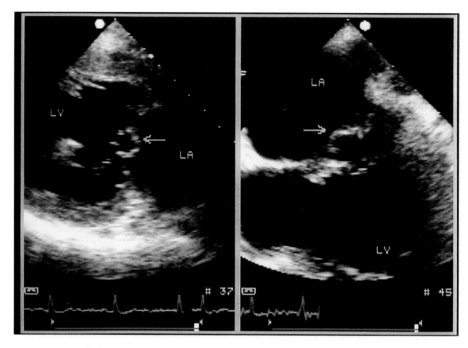

Fig. 12-16. Biplanar study from a patient with mitral valve prolapse, atrial fibrillation, and a history of stroke. *(Left)* Longitudinal transgastric two-chamber view showing a thickened mitral valve and prolapse of the posterior leaflet (arrow). *(Right)* Transverse four-chamber view demonstrating mitral valve prolapse (arrow). The left atrium (LA) is dilated. LV, left ventricle.

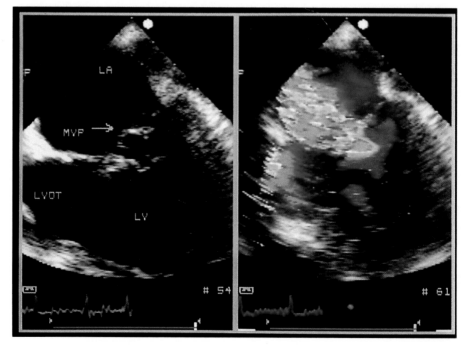

Fig. 12-17. Transverse five-chamber view of same patient shown in Figure 12-16. *(Left)* Mitral valve prolapse (MVP). *(Right)* Moderate eccentric mitral regurgitation on color Doppler. LA, left atrium; LV, left ventricle; LVOT, left ventricular outflow tract.

MITRAL VALVE PROLAPSE

Postmortem studies in patients with myxomatous valve involvement described endocardial friction lesions and platelet-fibrin deposits between the posterior mitral leaflet and the left atrial wall.[40,41] In addition, these lesions were found in conjunction with ischemic stroke.[42,43] Valvular fibrosis and thickening are common signs, and fissures of the valve surface are another nidus for thrombus formation.[44] In connection with these pathologic findings, it seem plausible that, with increasing histologic changes of the mitral valve apparatus, the likelihood of endocardial friction lesions and fibrin-platelet deposits in the mitral valve area increases.

TEE in young patients with cerebral ischemic events has shown a significantly higher incidence of mitral valve prolapse compared with a control group[45] (Figs. 12-16 and 12-17). TEE is also more sensitive in identifying a subgroup of patients with mitral valve prolapse who have thickened mitral valve leaflets.[45] Mitral regurgitation, rupture chordae tendineae, and cerebral ischemic events are more likely to develop in these patients.

LEFT VENTRICULAR APICAL THROMBI

Left ventricular apical thrombi in association with aneurysm and dilated cardiomyopathy are usually well evaluated by TTE.[46] The left ventricular apex, where most thrombi are located, is usually foreshortened by TEE using the transverse plane. However, the left ventricular apex is consistently visualized with use of the transgastric longitudinal view. Biplane TEE should be reserved for selected patients with suspected apical thrombi with technically difficult and nondiagnostic transthoracic images.

PROTRUDING ATHEROSCLEROTIC PLAQUE IN THE THORACIC AORTA

Biplane TEE imaging of the descending thoracic aorta and transverse aortic arch have permitted the detection of various degrees of atheromatous change, including intimal thickening, thrombus, penetrating atheromatous ulcer, intimal hematoma, and mobile projections from the atheromas, which move freely with the blood stream (Figs. 12-18 to 12-23). Several studies have reported a significant incidence of em-

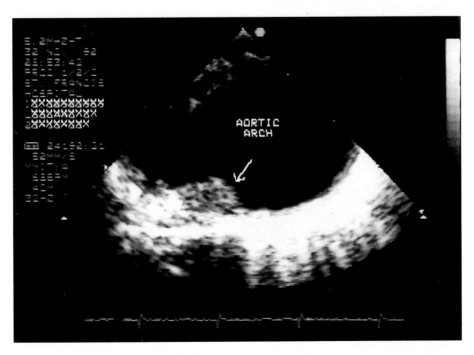

Fig. 12-18. Transverse view of the aortic arch showing a protruding atheroma (arrow) in a patient with cerebral emboli.

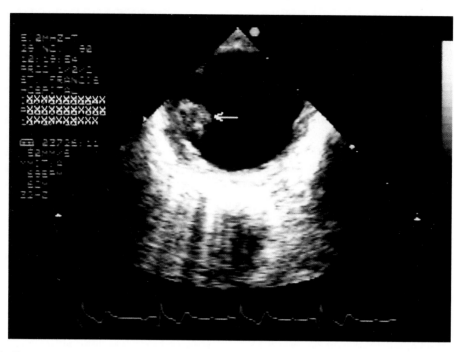

Fig. 12-19. Transverse view of the descending thoracic aorta demonstrating a protruding atheroma (arrow).

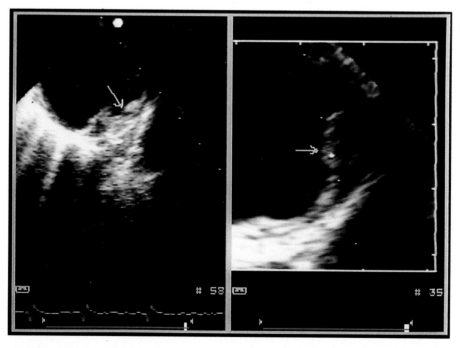

Fig. 12-20. *(Left)* Transverse view of an ulcerated lesion (arrow) in the descending aorta. *(Right)* Magnified view of the atheromatous ulcer (arrow).

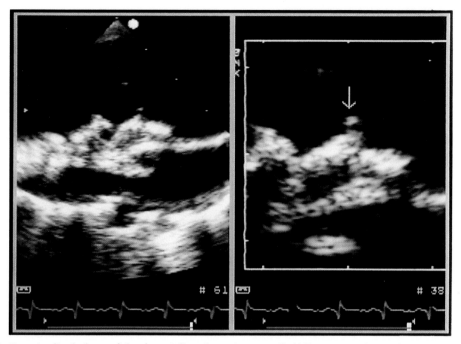

Fig. 12-21. Longitudinal plane of the descending thoracic aorta. *(Left)* Extensive atherosclerotic changes of the aorta with ulceration. *(Right)* Magnified view of small mobile lesion (arrow).

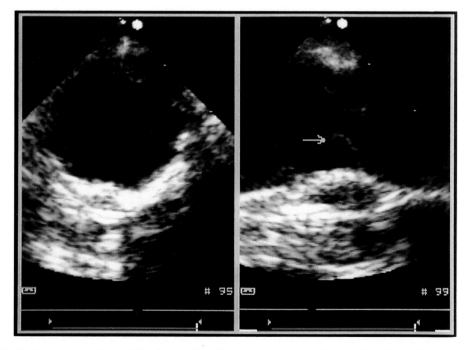

Fig. 12-22. Biplane examination of the descending thoracic aorta in a patient with peripheral systemic emboli. *(Left)* Transverse plane showing various degrees of atheromatous change. *(Right)* Longitudinal plane showing a mobile component (arrow) to the atheroma.

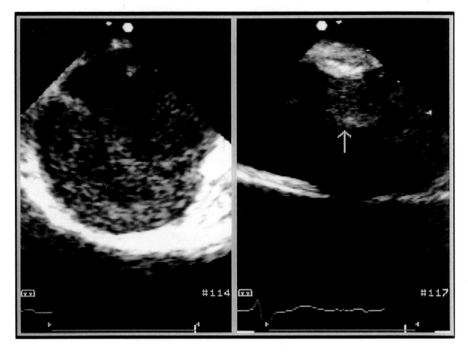

Fig. 12-23. Biplane imaging of the descending thoracic aorta. *(Left)* Transverse plane showing marked spontaneous echo contrast ("smoke") and atherosclerotic changes. *(Right)* Longitudinal plane revealing a large thrombus (arrow).

bolic events in patients with such lesions and an even higher rate of prior embolization in patients with mobile components to their atheromas.[47-49]

We have observed protruding atheromas with a mobile component in the transverse aortic arch in patients with cerebral ischemic events with normal carotid arterial studies and without an intracardiac source of emboli.

OTHER CARDIAC LESIONS

TEE is frequently helpful in the diagnosis of clots and vegetations associated with mechanical prosthesis, some of which may be responsible for systemic embolization. The high resolution obtainable with TEE also makes it possible to see small clots on the atrial surface of mechanical prostheses, which are also masked on TTE and which may be a source of embolization.

The transesophageal approach is also superior to TTE for the detection of vegetations in patients with native valves, which may be a source of emboli. TEE is especially helpful in diagnosing vegetations in unusual locations, such as on the mitral annulus[50] or on a left atrial myxoma.[51]

REFERENCES

1. Asinger RW. Cardiogenic brain embolism: the second report of the Cerebral Embolism Task Force. Arch Neurol 1989; 46:727–734.
2. Daniel W, Angermann C, Engerbending R, et al. Transesophageal echocardiography in patients with cerebral ischemic events and arterial embolism—a European Multicenter Study. Circulation 1989; 80(II):1883.
3. Wallach JB, Lukash L, Angrist AA. An interpretation of the incidence of mural thrombi in the left auricle and appendage with particular reference to mitral commissurotomy. Am Heart J 1953; 45:252–254.
4. Shrestha NA, Moreno FL, Narciso FV, et al. Two-dimensional echocardiographic diagnosis of left atrial thrombus in rheumatic heart disease. A clinicopathologic study. Circulation 1983; 67:341–347.

5. Meltzer RS, Visser CA, Fuster V. Intracardiac thrombi and systemic embolization. Ann Intern Med 1986; 104:689–698.
6. Aschenberg W, Schlüter M, Kremer P, et al. Transesophageal two-dimensional echocardiography for the detection of left atrial appendage thrombus. J Am Coll Cardiol 1986; 7:163–166.
7. Pollick C, Taylor D. Assessment of left atrial appendage function by transesophageal echocardiography. Implications for the development of thrombus. Circulation 1991; 84:223–231.
8. Kronzon I. Transesophageal echocardiography to detect atrial clots in candidates for percutaneous transseptal mitral balloon valvuloplasty. J Am Coll Cardiol 1990; 16:1320–1326.
9. Kronzon I. Transesophageal echocardiography during percutaneous mitral valvuloplasty. J Am Soc Echocardiogr 1989; 2:380–387.
10. Block PC. Early results of mitral balloon valvuloplasty for mitral stenosis: report from the NHLBI registry (abstract). Circulation 1989; 78(II):489.
11. Iliceto S, Antonelli G, Sorino M, et al. Dynamic intracavitary left atrial echoes in mitral stenosis. Am J Cardiol 1985; 55:603–606.
12. Chia BL, Choo MH, Yan PC, et al. Intra-atrial smoke-like echoes and thrombi formation. Chest 1989; 95:912–914.
13. Beppu S, Nimura Y, Sakakibara H, et al. Smoke-like echo in the left atrial cavity in mitral valve disease: its features and significance. J Am Coll Cardiol 1985; 6:744–749.
14. Erbel R, Stern H, Ehrenthal W, et al. Detection of spontaneous echocardiographic contrast within the left atrium by transesophageal echocardiography: spontaneous echocardiographic contrast. Clin Cardiol 1986; 9:245–252.
15. Daniel WG, Nellessen U, Schröder E, et al. Left atrial spontaneous echo contrast in mitral valve disease: an indicator for an increased thromboembolic risk. J Am Coll Cardiol 1988; 11:1204–1211.
16. Castello R, Pearson AC, Labovitz. Prevalence and clinical implications of atrial spontaneous contrast in patients undergoing transesophageal echocardiography. Am J Cardiol 1990; 65:1149–1153.
17. Chen YT, Kan MN, Chen JS, et al. Contributing factors to formation of left atrial spontaneous echo contrast in mitral valvular disease. J Ultrasound Med 1990; 9:151–155.
18. Black IW, Hopkins AP, Lee LCL, et al. Left atrial spontaneous echo contrast: a clinical and echocardiographic analysis. J Am Coll Cardiol 1991; 18:398–404.
19. Mahony C, Sublett KL, Harrison MR. Resolution of spontaneous contrast with platelet disaggregating therapy (Trifluperazine). Am J Cardiol 1989; 63:1009–1010.
20. De Belder MA, Tourikis L, Leech G, et al. Spontaneous contrast echoes are markers of thromboembolic risk in patients with atrial fibrillation. Circulation 1989; 80(suppl II):4.
21. Matsuzaki M, Toma Y, Suetsugu M, et al. Analysis of blood flow velocity and thrombogenesis in left atrial appendage by transesophageal two-dimensional echocardiography. J Am Coll Cardiol 1987; 9(suppl):21A.
22. Suetsugu M, Matsuzaki M, Toma Y, et al. Detection of mural thrombi and analysis of blood flow velocities in the left atrial appendage using transesophageal two-dimensional echocardiography and pulsed Doppler flowmetry. J Cardiol 1988; 18:385–394.
23. Matsuzaki M, Toma Y, Kusakawa R. Clinical applications of transesophageal echocardiography. Circulation 1990; 82: 709–722.
24. Thompson T, Evans W. Paradoxical embolism. Q J Med 1930; 23:135–150.
25. Harvey JA, Teague SM, Anderson JL, et al. Clinically silent atrial septal defects with evidence for cerebral embolization. Ann Intern Med 1986; 105:695–697.
26. Strunk BL, Cheitlin MD, Stulbarg MS, Schiller NB. Right-to-left interatrial shunting through a patent foramen ovale despite normal intracardiac pressures. Am J Cardiol 1987; 60:413–415.
27. Mügge A, Daniel WG, Klöpper JW, Lichtlen PR. Visualization of patent foramen ovale by transesophageal color-coded Doppler echocardiography. Am J Cardiol 1988; 62:837–838.
28. Khanderia BK. Prevalence of patent foramen ovale assessed by contrast transesophageal echocardiography. Circulation 1990; 82(III):109 (abst).
29. Langholz D, Louie EK, Konstadt SN, et al. Transesophageal echocardiographic demonstration of distinct mechanisms for right to left shunting across a patent foramen ovale in the absence of pulmonary hypertension. J Am Coll Cardiol 1991; 18:1112–1117.
30. Lang FJ, Posselt A. Aneurysmatische Vorwölburg der Fossa ovalis in den linken Vorhof. Wein Med Wochenschr 1934; 84:392–397.
31. Silver MD, Dorsey JS. Aneurysms of the septum primum in adults. Arch Pathol Lab Med 1978; 102:62–69.
32. Burstow DJ, McEmery PT, Stafford EG. Fenestrated atrial septal aneurysm: diagnosis by transesophageal echocardiography. J Am Soc Echocardiogr 1990; 3:500–504.
33. Anderson GJ, Swartz J. Two-dimensional echocardiographic recognition of an atrial septal aneurysm. Int J Cardiol 1983; 2:447–452.
34. Ong LS, Nanda NC, Falkoff M, et al. Interatrial septal aneurysm, systolic click and atrial tachyarrhythmias: a new syndrome? Ultrasound Med Biol 1982; 8:691–700.
35. Gondi B, Nanda N. Two-dimensional echocardiographic features of atrial septal aneurysms. Circulation 1981; 63:452–459.
36. Hanley PC, Tajik AJ, Hynes JK, et al. Diagnosis and classification of atrial septal aneurysms by two-dimensional echocardiography: report of 80 consecutive cases. J Am Coll Cardiol 1985; 6:1370–1378.
37. Chen TO. Atrial septal aneurysms as a "newly discovered" cause of stroke in patients with mitral valve prolapse. Am J Cardiol 1990; 67:327–331.
38. Zabalgoitia-Reyes M. A possible mechanism for neurologic ischemic events in patients with atrial septal aneurysm. Am J Cardiol 1990; 66:761–765.
39. Zboyovsky KL, Nanda NC, Jain H. Transesophageal echocardiographic identification of atrial septal aneurysm. Echocardiography 1991; 8:435–437.
40. Chester E, King RA, Edwards JE. The myxomatous mitral valve and sudden death. Circulation 1983; 67:632–639.
41. Lucas RV, Edwards JE. The floppy mitral valve. Curr Probl Cardiol 1982; 7:1–48.
42. Bramlet DA, Decker EL, Floyd WL. Nonbacterial thrombotic endocarditis as a cause of stroke in mitral valve prolapse. South Med J 1982; 75:1133–1135.
43. Schnee MA, Bucal AA. Fatal embolism in mitral valve prolapse. Chest 1983; 83:285–287.
44. Olsen EGJ, Al-Rufaie HK. The floppy mitral valve. Study on pathogenesis. Br Heart J 1980; 44:674–683.
45. Zenker G, Erbel R, Krämer G, et al. Transesophageal two-

dimensional echocardiography in young patients with cerebral ischemic events. Stroke 1988; 19:345–348.

46. Reeder GS, Tajik AJ, Seward JB. Left ventricular mural thrombus: two-dimensional echocardiographic diagnosis. Mayo Clin Proc 1981; 56:82–86.

47. Tunick PA, Kronzon I. Protruding atherosclerotic plaque in the aortic arch of patients with systemic embolization: a new finding seen by transesophageal echocardiography. Am Heart J 1990; 120:658–662.

48. Tunick PA, Kronzon I. The association between protruding plaques in the thoracic aorta and systemic embolization. J Am Coll Cardiol 1991; 17:261A (abst).

49. Tunick PA, Kronzon I. Transesophageal echocardiography in embolic disease. Cardio 1991; 7:72–85.

50. Tunick PA. Unusual mitral annular vegetation diagnosed by transesophageal echocardiography. Am Heart J 1990; 120:444–446.

51. Tunick PA. The echocardiographic recognition of an atrial myxoma vegetation. Am Heart J 1990; 119:679–681.

13 Coronary Artery Disease

IMAGING OF CORONARY ARTERIES

The imaging of a coronary artery by conventional precordial echocardiography has been reported, but the image quality is generally too poor to permit evaluation of the anatomic details in adult patients. High-resolution images of the proximal coronary artery can be obtained by the higher-frequency (5-MHz) transesophageal probe,[1] with an imaging quality superior to that of transthoracic recordings. The main trunk of the left coronary artery from the left coronary sinus and its bifurcation into the left anterior descending and circumflex coronary artery can frequently be visualized (see Ch. 4, Fig. 4-11). The right coronary artery is seen to originate from the right aortic sinus, usually at a tomographic level different from that of the left coronary artery, and detection of its image is much more difficult than that of the left coronary artery[2] (see Ch. 4, Fig. 4-12). A flow velocity signal, particularly in the left anterior descending, is often detectable by positioning the sample volume in the lumen; adjustment of the angle between the ultrasound beam and the flow direction is necessary to record a proper flow velocity by monitoring color Doppler flow images. The diastolic component of the signal can usually be obtained satisfactorily when the image of the left anterior descending is clearly demonstrated. However, the flow signal during systole is often not necessarily stable enough for analysis because of displacement of the sample volume by the abrupt systolic movement of the heart.

Recently, Yoshida et al.[3] reported that adequate images of the full length of the left main coronary artery and identification of the bifurcation of the left anterior descending and circumflex coronary artery were obtained in 60 of 67 patients (90 percent) by TEE. They also demonstrated quantitative evaluation of left main coronary artery narrowing (greater than 50 percent) in 10 of 11 patients (sensitivity, 91 percent) and insignificant narrowing or no abnormalities of the coronary lumen in the other 49 patients (specificity, 100 percent) (Figs. 13-1 and 13-2). The blood flow signal in the left main coronary artery was detected in 57 of 67 patients (85 percent) by the transesophageal color Doppler image. In their report, the positive and negative predictive accuracies for left main coronary artery disease were 100 percent and 98 percent, respectively. Yamagishi et al.[2] reported that TEE provided images of the left anterior descending in 77 percent of all patients examined, and a stable flow signal from the proximal left anterior descending could be recorded in all patients in whom the image of the left coronary artery was well visualized; however, the detection rate of the right coronary artery (26 percent) was much lower than that of

133

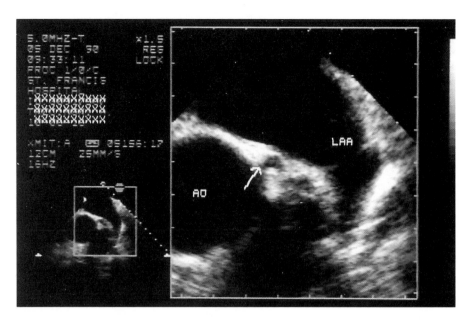

Fig. 13-1. Transverse basal short-axis view of the left main coronary artery. The arrow points to a severe ostial stenosis. Coronary arteriography revealed a critical left main coronary stenosis. AO, aorta; LAA, left atrial appendage.

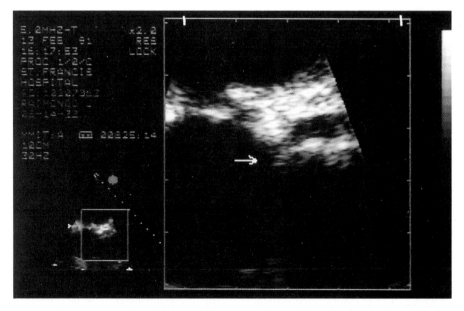

Fig. 13-2. Transverse basal short-axis view of a critical left main ostial coronary artery stenosis (arrow). TEE findings were confirmed by coronary arteriography.

the left coronary artery, and precise analysis of the right coronary flow pattern was not possible because of numerous noise signals. Schnittger et al.[4] visualized the left main coronary artery in 15 (75 percent) and the right coronary artery in 7 (35 percent) of 20 patients studied by TEE. Further study will be necessary to demonstrate the clinical value of TEE assessment of coronary arterial morphology and pathophysiology.

TEE should prove useful in evaluation of coronary artery aneurysms seen in patients with Kawasaki's disease. TEE has also been used to demonstrate atherosclerotic coronary artery aneurysms,[5] aortocoronary venous bypass graft aneurysm,[6] coronary arteriovenous fistula,[7] and coronary artery to coronary sinus fistula.[8] We have also recently reported a case of a left coronary artery to left ventricular fistula.[9]

MECHANICAL COMPLICATIONS OF ACUTE MYOCARDIAL INFARCTION

TEE has also been used in the evaluation of mechanical complications following acute myocardial infarction, such as ventricular septal rupture (Fig. 13-3) and papillary muscle rupture[10-12] (Figs. 13-4 and 13-5). In many instances, on the basis of TEE images, medical or surgical treatment can be instituted promptly without further diagnostic procedures or an invasive procedure limited to coronary arteriography. TEE is especially useful in patients with suboptimal and nondiagnostic thoracic images.

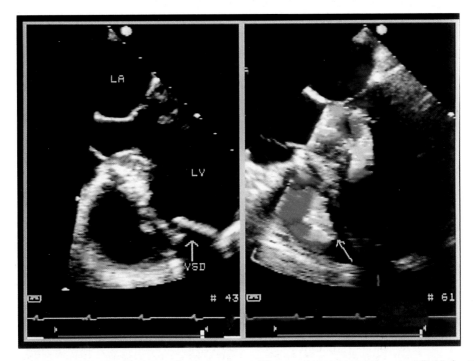

Fig. 13-3. Transverse four-chamber view from a patient with a recent anteroseptal myocardial infarction complicated by ventricular septal rupture in the apical region, requiring urgent surgery. *(Left)* Postoperative image showing the patch at the site of repair with findings of dehiscence and residual ventricular septal defect (VSD). *(Right)* Color Doppler showing a mosaic-colored signal of left-to-right shunt (arrow). LA, left atrium; LV, left ventricle.

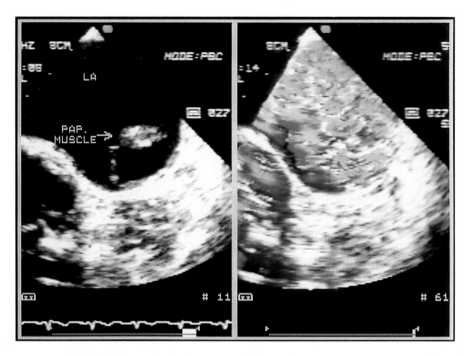

Fig. 13-4. Transverse basal short-axis view of posteromedial papillary muscle rupture. *(Left)* Head of papillary muscle (pap. muscle) prolapsing in the left atrium (LA). *(Right)* Color Doppler imaging of severe mitral regurgitation. The left atrium is totally opacified by a mosaic blue-green signal.

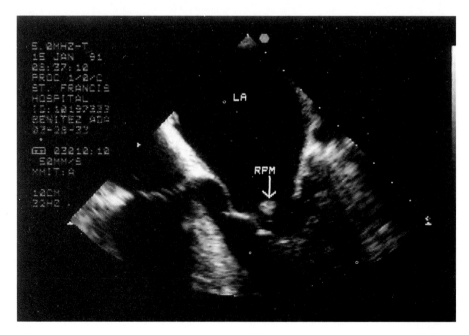

Fig. 13-5. Posteromedial papillary muscle rupture (RPM) following an inferior wall myocardial infarction. LA, left atrium.

EXERCISE TEE IN CORONARY ARTERY DISEASE

Exercise transthoracic 2-D echocardiography has proved useful in the diagnosis and management of patients with coronary artery disease, providing visualization of exercise-induced regional wall motion abnormalities. However, this technique does not always produce good images. The use of TEE during exercise provides some advantages, especially a better quality of imaging, but the patient's having to exercise with a TEE probe in place is a clear disadvantage. In those who cannot exercise, alternative methods of inducing myocardial ischemia that would permit the use of TEE include dobutamine infusion, intravenous dipyridamole testing, and combined imaging and esophageal pacing.

REFERENCES

1. Zwicky P, Daniel WG, Mügge A, Lichtlen PR. Imaging of coronary arteries by color-coded transesophageal Doppler echocardiography. Am J Cardiol 1988; 62:639–640.
2. Yamagishi N, Nimura Y. Assessment of coronary blood flow by transesophageal two-dimensional pulsed Doppler echocardiography. Am J Cardiol 1988; 65:641–644.
3. Yoshida K, Yoshikawa J, Hozumi T, et al. Detection of left main coronary artery stenosis by transesophageal color Doppler and two-dimensional echocardiography. Circulation 1990; 81:1271–1276.
4. Schnittger I, Nellessen U, Appleton C, Popp RL. Visualization of coronary arteries and detection of coronary arteries and detection of coronary blood flows using transesophageal echocardiography. J Am Coll Cardiol 1988; 11:152A (abst).
5. Tunick PA, Slater J, Pasternack P, Kronzon I. Coronary artery aneurysms: A transesophageal echocardiographic study. Am Heart J 1989; 118:176–179.
6. Dzavik V, Lamay M, Chan RL. Echocardiographic diagnosis of an aortocoronary venous bypass graft aneurysm. Am Heart J 1989; 118:619–621.
7. Calafiore PA, Raymond R, Schiavone WA, Rosenkranz ER. Precise evaluation of a complex coronary arteriovenous fistula: the utility of transesophageal color Doppler. J Am Soc Echocardiogr 1989; 2:337–341.
8. Samdarshi TE, Mahan EF III, Nanda NC, Sanyal RS. Transesophageal echocardiographic assessment of congenital coronary artery to coronary sinus fistulas in adults. Am J Cardiol 1991; 68:263–266.
9. Mian MS, Freund T, Missri JC. Left coronary to left ventricular fistula: angiographic and transesophageal echocardiographic features. J Cardiovasc Technol 1991; 10:45–48.
10. Koenig K, Kasper W, Hofmann T, et al. Transesophageal echocardiography for diagnosis of rupture of the ventricular septum or left ventricular papillary muscle during acute myocardial infarction. Am J Cardiol 1987; 59:362.
11. Oh JK, Seward JB, Khandheria BK. Transesophageal echocardiography in the intensive care unit. Circulation 1988; 78(suppl II):298 (abst).
12. Patel AM, Miller FA, Khandheria BK, et al. Role of transesophageal echocardiography in the diagnosis of papillary muscle rupture secondary to myocardial infarction. Am Heart J 1989; 118:1330–1333.

14 Evaluation of Congenital Heart Disease in the Adult

TEE may be an important adjunct in the evaluation of patients with repaired and unrepaired congenital heart disease. Atrial and ventricular septal defects can be directly visualized, and shunt flow can be confirmed by color Doppler and contrast echocardiography.[1,2] Color Doppler and saline contrast can be used to delineate the extent and timing of left-to-right and right-to-left shunting. High-resolution images of the interatrial septum permit the differentiation of sinus venosus from secundum or primum atrial septal defects. In patients with Ebstein's anomaly, TEE helps define tricuspid valve pathology as well as possible associated interatrial shunting. Furthermore, diseases of the aorta, such as coarctation, can be clearly demonstrated by TEE.

In the operating room, TEE is accepted as an important adjunct to assist the surgeon in determining the adequacy of such procedures as repair of atrial or ventricular septal defects. Echo contrast, color Doppler, and Doppler echocardiographic imaging are used to assess valvular competence as well as residual shunting.

Although intraoperative epicardial imaging has been established as a powerful method to assess the adequacy of surgical repair and to evaluate left ventricular function, a major advantage of TEE is that it does not interfere with the operating field and thus permits continuous monitoring of cardiac function.

TEE is not restricted to the adult patient population. A specially designed pediatric transesophageal probe (Aloka) has been developed for use with the Aloka SSD 870 ultrasound system. The ultrasound transducer, mounted on a pediatric bronchoscope with a shaft diameter of 6 mm and a maximal tip dimension of 7×8 mm (24 elements, frequency 5 MHz), permits cross-sectional imaging, color Doppler mapping, and pulsed wave Doppler investigation. Studies have been done in infants and children ranging from 1 year to 14 years, including patients weighing less than 15 kg.[3] This has permitted the use of TEE in infants and children for the assessment of some selected complex congenital lesions.

This chapter focuses on the most common congenital heart lesions seen in the adult. Included are atrial septal defects (ASDs), ventricular septal defects (VSDs), Ebstein's anomaly, and persistent left superior vena cava. Further details and discussion of less common entities are available in more specialized textbooks dealing specifically with congenital heart disease.[4-6]

ATRIAL SEPTAL DEFECT

Atrial septal defect accounts for approximately 25 percent of congenital heart lesions seen in the adult.[4] Patients who have eluded earlier diagnosis as well as those who have undergone prior correction of the defect may present for echocardiographic evaluation. Women with this disorder outnumber men by 3:1.

Anatomy

The size and contour of the defect are variable. Defects are classified as secundum (70 percent), primum or partial atrioventricular canal (15 percent), and sinus venosus types (15 percent). These classifications are based on the location of the defect within the septum: in the region of the fossa ovalis, the AV junction, or the posterior septum, respectively. This classification system is useful because each type has different associated anomalies: one-third of secundum defects have associated mitral valve prolapse, two-thirds of primum defects have a cleft anterior mitral valve leaflet, and one-half of sinus venosus defects have anomalous drainage of the right pulmonary veins.

Echocardiography

Although transthoracic echo-Doppler examination is excellent in diagnosing more than 95 percent of ostium secundum and nearly 100 percent of ostium primum defects, evaluation of sinus venosus ASDs is less satisfactory.[7] Since TEE can visualize the entire atrial septum, this technique should be able to detect all ASDs, regardless of location.

Biplane TEE can reliably differentiate ostium secundum, ostium primum, and sinus venosus ASDs and permits evaluation of partial anomalous pulmonary venous return, which is frequently associated with the latter lesion.[8] The direct connection of the right upper pulmonary vein to the right atrium can be clearly visualized. Views of the atrial septum in particular, the valve of the fossa ovalis and the superior and inferior limbi of the atrial septum, are optimally obtained with the longitudinal array. Patent foramen ovale (see Ch. 12) and sinus venosus defects are imaged better with the biplanar than with the single-plane examination. In our laboratory, we combine color Doppler flow mapping and intravenous agitated saline contrast injection to assess patients with suspected ASDs (Figs. 14-1 to 14-8) and patent foramen ovale. The size of the defect in the atrial septum from the transesophageal approach has been found to correlate well with direct measurement during cardiac surgery, and a high linear correlation was obtained between shunt flow volumes across the defect and that obtained by the Fick method.[9]

Recently, Yoshida et al.[10] reported the assessment of left-to-right atrial shunting after percutaneous mitral valvuloplasty by TEE. On the first day after valvulo-

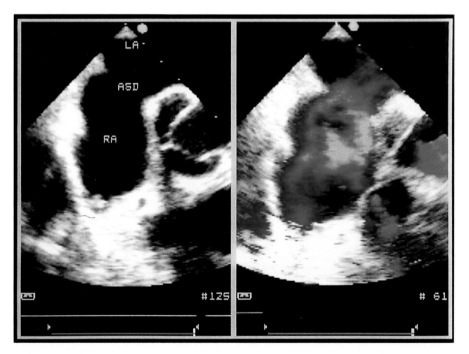

Fig. 14-1. *(Left)* Transverse basal short-axis view of a large ostium secundum atrial septal defect (ASD). *(Right)* Color Doppler image of left-to-right shunt across the ASD. LA, left atrium; RA, right atrium.

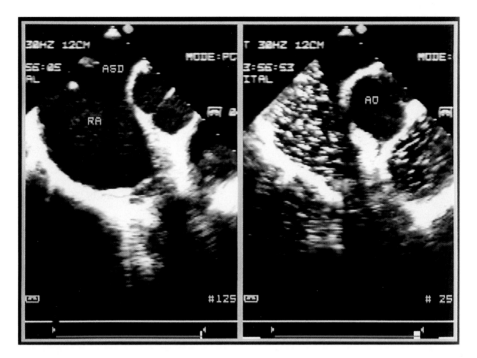

Fig. 14-2. *(Left)* Secundum atrial septal defect (ASD). The right atrium (RA) is enlarged *(Right)* Agitated saline contrast injection demonstrates microbubbles in the RA and a negative contrast image caused by displacement of the microbubbles from left-to-right shunt. AO, aorta.

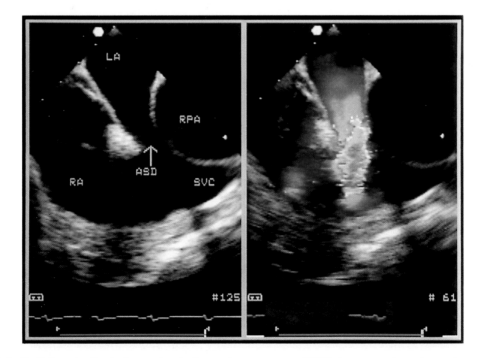

Fig. 14-3. *(Left)* Longitudinal view at level of superior vena cava (SVC) demonstrating a large sinus venosus atrial septal defect (ASD). *(Right)* Color Doppler showing flow across the defect from left atrium (LA) to right atrium (RA). The right pulmonary artery (RPA) is enlarged.

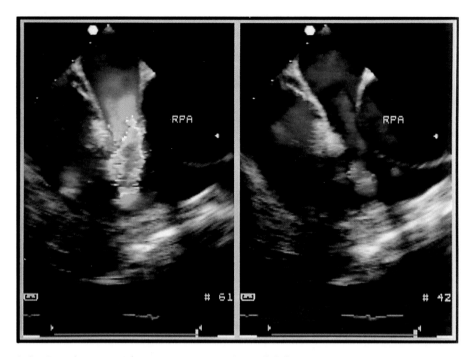

Fig. 14-4. Color Doppler image of sinus venosus atrial septal defect, same patient as shown in Figure 14-3. A bidirectional shunt is recorded. *(Left)* Left-to-right shunt. *(Right)* Right-to-left shunt. RPA, right pulmonary artery.

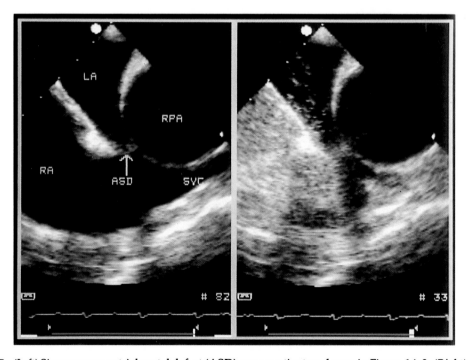

Fig. 14-5. *(Left)* Sinus venosus atrial septal defect (ASD), same patient as shown in Figure 14-3. *(Right)* Agitated saline contrast study demonstrating microbubbles in the left atrium (LA) and a negative contrast study at the junction of the superior vena cava (SVC) and right atrium (RA), findings consistent with a bidirectional shunt. RPA, right pulmonary artery.

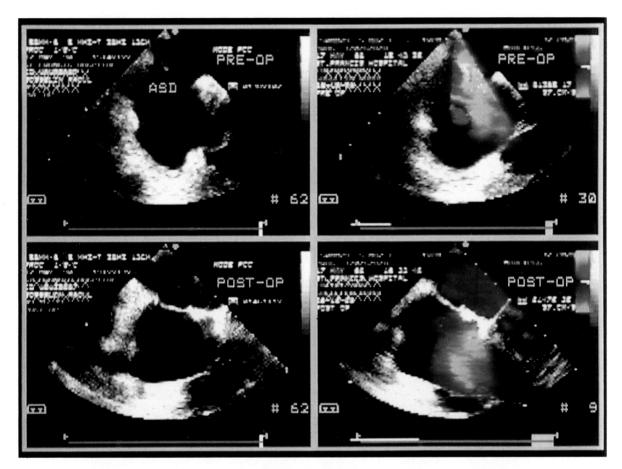

Fig. 14-6. Intraoperative study of patient with secundum atrial septal defect (ASD). *(Upper left)* Preoperative study showing a large ASD. *(Upper right)* Color Doppler image of left-to-right shunt. *(Lower left)* Postoperative study following closure of ASD. *(Lower right)* Color Doppler image without residual shunt.

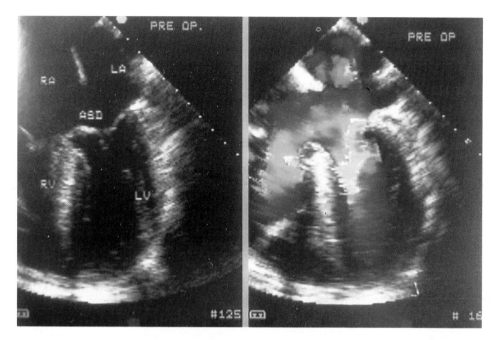

Fig. 14-7. *(Left)* Preoperative study in the transverse four-chamber view of patient with ostium primum atrial septal defect (ASD). *(Right)* Color Doppler showing a left-to-right shunt across the ASD. LA, left atrium; LV, left ventricle; RA, right atrium; RV, right ventricle.

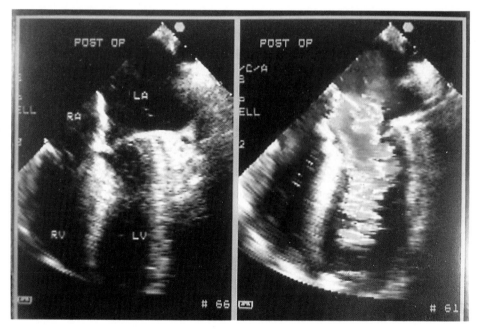

Fig. 14-8. Postoperative study, same patient as shown in Figure 14-7. *(Left)* Closure of ostium primum atrial septal defect with patch. *(Right)* Normal color Doppler study. There is no residual shunt. LA, left atrium; LV, left ventricle; RA, right atrium; RV, right ventricle.

plasty, transesophageal color Doppler echocardiography demonstrated atrial shunts in 13 of 15 patients (87 percent) without a significant oxygen step-up. The mean diameter of the ASD detected by TEE was 1.8 ± 1.0 mm. Six months after valvuloplasty, however, the shunt flow remained in only three patients (20 percent) and was associated with a significant decrease in the diameter of the atrial defect.

We do not recommend TEE as a routine examination in the assessment of ASD, but we suggest that it is indicated in patients with inadequate or nondiagnostic results by the transthoracic approach.

VENTRICULAR SEPTAL DEFECT

Although ventricular septal defect (VSD) occurs in almost 1 in 500 normal births, nearly 50 percent close spontaneously during childhood; thus, in adults it is less common and accounts for approximately 12 percent of congenital heart abnormalities seen in adults. Adult patients presenting to the physician include those with small inconsequential defects, those who have undergone prior palliative or corrective surgical procedures, and those with acquired complications.

Anatomy

Ventricular septal defects are classified according to the location within the interventricular septum. Seventy percent are membranous defects involving the pars membranacea. They are variably sized and shaped and often close spontaneously. Muscular defects occur within the muscular portion of the septum, toward the apex, and within the mid- and posterior regions. Multiple defects may be present and also often close spontaneously. In both circumstances, associated cardiac defects are uncommon. AV canal defects involve the posterobasal septum, are usually large, and are associated with mitral and tricuspid valve clefts, as well as with a primum-type ASD. These are common in patients with Down's syndrome. Supracristal (subaortic) defects are uncommon (5 percent). They are usually small; however, their strategic location beneath the aortic annulus may undermine aortic leaflet support and may cause progressive aortic incompetence.

Echocardiography

Ventricular septal defects can also be diagnosed by TEE (Fig. 14-9). However, the experience is less than

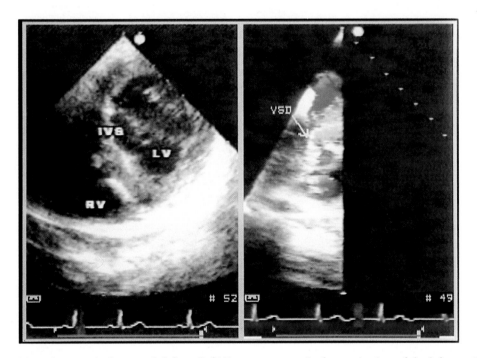

Fig. 14-9. Muscular ventricular septal defect. *(Left)* Transverse gastric short-axis view of the left ventricle (LV) demonstrating discontinuity of the interventricular septum (IVS). *(Right)* Color Doppler demonstrating a mosaic color jet of left-to-right across the ventricular septal defect (VSD). The defect was not visualized on transthoracic study. RV, right ventricle.

that for ASDs. Biplanar imaging measurably enhances the visualization of the ventricular septum. Apical, small, or multiple VSDs are also easily diagnosed using biplane imaging.

At present, 2-D echocardiography and Doppler examination are usually diagnostic in most patients. They delineate the presence, size, and location of VSDs, and the presence of associated cardiac lesions and secondary problems, including right ventricular or pulmonary artery hypertension. TEE should be reserved for patients in whom a VSD is suspected but the transthoracic images are inadequate or nondiagnostic.

EBSTEIN'S ANOMALY

Transthoracic echocardiography is useful in the evaluation of Ebstein's anomaly; however, resolution of certain structures are sometimes suboptimal. Because of its posterior positioning and proximity to the heart, TEE can often achieve higher-quality and more detailed images of the posterior structures, as well as the right-sided chambers and tricuspid valve. The characteristic findings of Ebstein's anomaly, as seen by TEE, include a large "sail-like" anterior leaflet and apically displaced septal and inferior leaflets.[11] An enlarged right atrium and ventricle can be demonstrated with the right ventricle divided into proximal and distal chambers by the tricuspid valve. Color Doppler imaging usually demonstrates tricuspid regurgitation with the regurgitant jet originating from the tricuspid valve coaptation point in the distal right ventricular chamber. Several individual regurgitant jet can be identified through fenestrations in the distal anterior leaflet (Fig. 14-10).

Other associated congenital anomalies include ASD (Fig. 14-11), pulmonic stenosis, and pulmonary outflow aneurysmal dilation. With the advent of biplane TEE, it is now possible to evaluate the right ventricular outflow tract and pulmonic valve.

TEE is useful intraoperatively to assess the anatomical and functional results of surgery[11,12] (Fig. 14-12). This includes closure of associated ASD, as well as

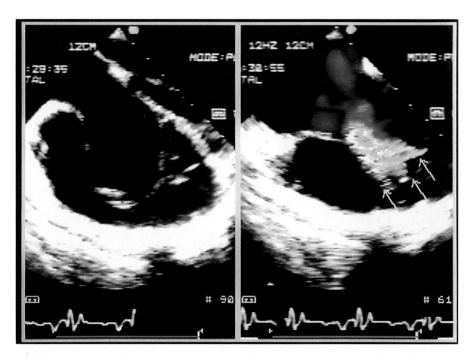

Fig. 14-10. Ebstein's anomaly of the tricuspid valve. *(Left)* Transverse two-chamber view of the right cardiac chambers showing an elongated, "sail-like" anterior leaflet and an apically displaced septal leaflet dividing the right ventricle into proximal and distal chambers. The anterior leaflet is shown to be attached to the annulus. *(Right)* Color Doppler demonstrating multiple tricuspid regurgitant jets (arrows). These jets originate from the tricuspid valve coaptation point and from anterior leaflet fenestrations.

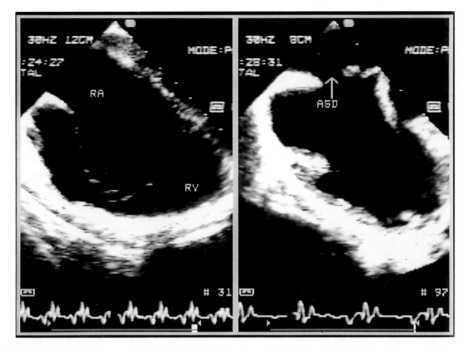

Fig. 14-11. *(Left)* Ebstein's anomaly of the tricuspid valve. *(Right)* Associated secundum atrial septal defect (ASD). RA, right atrium; RV, right ventricle.

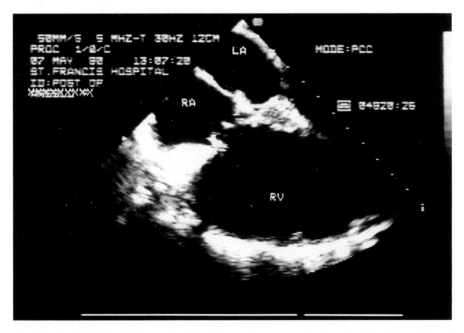

Fig. 14-12. Transverse midesophageal view of the right atrium (RA) and right ventricle (RV) following surgical correction of Ebstein's anomaly of the tricuspid valve with a Duran annuloplasty ring.

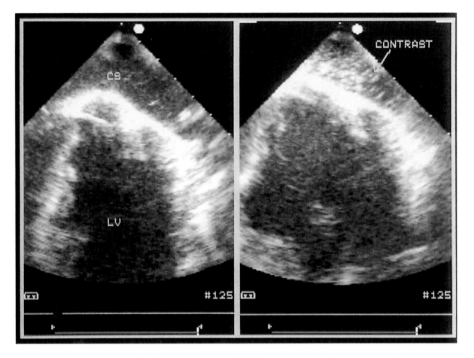

Fig. 14-13. Transverse view at level of coronary sinus (CS) in a patient with persistent left superior vena cava. *(Left)* The CS is dilated. *(Right)* Injection of agitated saline contrast from a left antecubital vein revealing microbubbles in the CS. LV, left ventricle.

assessment of the degree of postoperative tricuspid regurgitation. Echocardiographic evaluation of anterior tricuspid leaflet mobility is important in predicting the outcome of annuloplasty.[12] Successful operative repair depends on a mobile normal-sized or enlarged anterior leaflet that is not complete tethered and shows large excursion. A restrictive and tethered anterior leaflet or a small functional right ventricle usually predicts the need for valve replacement. Thus, TEE is important in the diagnosis of Ebstein's anomaly and in the evaluation of its operative repair.

OTHER CONGENITAL HEART DISEASES

Other congenital heart diseases in which TEE has a role include subaortic membrane,[13,14] left atrial membrane and cor triatriatum,[15,16] supramitral ring and parachute mitral valve, and visualization and flow characterization of certain anomalous vessels, such as the left superior vena cava (Fig. 14-13) and the azygos vein.[17] Bicuspid aortic valve with aortic regurgitation and mitral valve prolapse are dealt with in Chapters 5 and 6, respectively. Coronary artery fistulas are discussed in Chapter 13.

REFERENCES

1. Cyran SE, Kimball TR, Meyer RA, et al. Efficacy of intraoperative transesophageal echocardiography in children with congenital heart disease. Am J Cardiol 1989; 63:594–598.
2. Hanrath P, Schlüter M, Langenstein BA, et al. Detection of ostium secundum atrial septal defects by transesophageal cross-sectional echocardiography. Br Heart J 1983; 49:350–358.
3. Stümper OFW, Elzenga NJ, Hess J, Sutherland GR. Transesophageal echocardiography in children with congenital heart disease: an initial experience.
4. Liberthson RR. Congenital Heart Disease Diagnosis and Management in Children and Adults. Boston: Little, Brown, 1989.
5. Perloff J. The Clinical Recognition of Congenital Heart Disease, (3rd Ed.) Philadelphia: WB Saunders, 1987.
6. Roberts WC. Adult Congenital Heart Disease. Philadelphia: FA Davis, 1987.
7. Shub C, Dimopoulos IN, Seward JB, et al. Sensitivity of two-dimensional echocardiography in the direct visualization of

atrial septal defect utilizing the subcostal approach: experience with 154 patients. J Am Coll Cardiol 1983; 2:127–135.

8. Seward JB, Khandheria BK, Edwards WD, et al. Biplanar transesophageal echocardiography: anatomic correlations, image orientation, and clinical applications. Mayo Clin Proc 1990; 65:1193–1213.

9. Morimoto K, Matsuzaki M, Tohma Y, et al. Atrial septal defect diagnosed and quantitatively-evaluated by transesophageal two-dimensional Doppler echocardiography. J Cardiol 1988; 18:813–822.

10. Yoshida K, Yoshikawa J, Akasaka T, et al. Assessment of left-to-right atrial shunting after percutaneous mitral valvuloplasty by transesophageal color Doppler flow-mapping. Circulation 1989; 80:1521–1526.

11. Fram DB, Missri J, Therrien ML, Chawla S. Assessment of Ebstein's anomaly and to surgical repair using transesophageal two-dimensional echocardiography and Doppler color flow mapping. Echocardiography 1991; 8:367–371.

12. Shüna A, Seward JB, Tajik AJ. Two-dimensional echocardiographic-surgical correlation in Ebstein's anomaly: preopera-

tive determination of patients requiring tricuspid valve plication versus replacement. Circulation 1983; 68:534–541.

13. Mügge A, Daniel WG, Wolpers HG, et al. Improved visualization of discrete subvalvular aortic stenosis by transesophageal color-coded Doppler echocardiography. Am Heart J 1989; 117:474–475.

14. Schwinger ME, Kronzon I. Improved evaluation of left ventricular outflow tract obstruction by transesophageal echocardiography. J Am Soc Echocardiogr 1989; 2:191–193.

15. Goldfarb A, Weinreb J, Daniel WG, Kronzon I. A patient with right and left atrial membranes: the role of transesophageal echocardiography and magnetic resonance imaging in diagnosis. J Am Soc Echocardiogr 1989; 2:350–353.

16. Schlüter M, Langenstein BA, Thier W, et al. Transesophageal two-dimensional echocardiography in the diagnosis of cor triatriatum in the adult. J Am Coll Cardiol 1983; 2:1011–1015.

17. Sukigara M, Komazaki T, Ohata M, et al. Transesophageal real-time two-dimensional Doppler echography: a new method for the evaluation of azygos venous flow. Gastrointest Endosc 1988; 34:125–127.

15 Transesophageal Echocardiography in Critically Ill Patients

Echocardiography has evolved into a procedure that is unmatched in terms of the versatility and variety of information that is provided and is therefore ideal for the evaluation of critically ill patients. Cardiac emergencies may be encountered anywhere in the hospital, in the emergency department, intensive care unit (ICU), cardiac catheterization laboratory, or the operating room. The emergency may be caused by acute exacerbation or complications of a previously unrecognized chronic disease or by the acute onset of a new disorder. In a cardiac emergency, abnormalities such as a new murmur on physical examination, acute ischemic changes on the electrocardiogram (ECG), pulmonary vascular congestion or an enlarged cardiac silhouette on the chest radiograph, or a new rise in myocardial enzymes warrant rapid clarification. The successful use of echocardiography requires a thorough understanding of the various cardiac disorders that can result in emergency situations and an adept ability to delineate the echocardiographic manifestations of these disorders.

The value of transthoracic echocardiography (TTE) is frequently limited in these critically ill patients, who may be on life-support devices or who may have recent surgical wounds restricting the transthoracic imaging windows. Such external constraints do not interfere with TEE. Although it is semi-invasive, the TEE procedure is well tolerated by most critically ill patients, some of whom may be in cardiogenic shock.[1] However, TEE may aggravate hemodynamic instability of the critically ill patient and should be performed by a physician-echocardiographer who can handle cardiac emergencies. Table 15-1 lists the most frequent indications for emergency TEE in our institution. We have found TEE particularly useful in diagnosing complications of acute myocardial infarction, such as papillary muscle rupture, ventricular septal defect, right ventricular infarction, and ventricular aneurysms or pseudoaneurysms. In addition, this technique is useful in evaluating potential donor hearts for cardiac transplantation, in immediate postoperative hypotensive crisis, and in patients in a state of shock. It is also valuable in critical aortic stenosis that cannot be diagnosed owing to inadequate transthoracic images, aortic dissection, acute infective endocarditis, and prosthetic valve dysfunction. On the basis of information obtained by TEE, medical or surgical treatment can be instituted promptly without further diagnostic procedures[2]; in some cases, negative TEE examinations can also confidently exclude a suspected diagnosis.

Table 15-1. Indications for Emergency TEE in 120 Patients

Indication	Total	(%)
Source of embolus	22	18
Acute native valve dysfunction	20	17
Vegetations, abscess	17	14
Ventricular dysfunction	15	13
Complications of myocardial infarction	12	10
Aortic dissection	12	10
Prosthetic valve dysfunction	10	8
Chest trauma	5	4
Cardiac tamponade	5	4
Potential donor hearts	2	2

This chapter reviews the value of TEE in critically ill patients. Most of the topics have been previously discussed; the corresponding chapters are listed next to each subheading.

NATIVE AND PROSTHETIC VALVE DYSFUNCTION

TEE has been shown to be extremely helpful in the recognition and characterization of mitral valve pathology, such as ruptured chordae tendineae and flail leaflets.[3,4] Furthermore, several investigators have reported superior accuracy, sensitivity, and reliability of TEE over TTE for mitral prosthetic dysfunction, for which ultrasonic shadowing of the left atrium frequently occurs with the standard surface studies[5-7] (see Chs. 6 and 8).

Our experience is in agreement with previous observations that TEE is more sensitive than TTE for detection of mitral valve regurgitation. We have found TTE to underestimate the severity of mitral regurgitation, particularly with eccentric jets and in patients with prosthetic valve regurgitation.

INFECTIVE ENDOCARDITIS

Echocardiography is the diagnostic procedure of choice for the noninvasive diagnosis of endocarditis (see Ch. 10). TEE is superior to TTE in the detection of valvular vegetations[8] and the characterization of certain complications of endocarditis, including regurgitation of the valve, ring abscesses, sinus of Valsalva and mycotic aneurysms, subaortic aneurysm from mitral-aortic intervalvular fibrosa and rupture of subaortic aneurysm into the left atrium.

In many instances, surgery is performed solely on the basis of information derived from TEE, avoiding cardiac catheterization.

CARDIAC SOURCES OF EMBOLIZATION

The most frequent source of cardiac embolization is a thrombus in the left atrial appendage, which cannot be visualized using the transthoracic approach (see Ch. 12). With TEE, this structure is easily visualized.

Because of the great depth using the apical or parasternal approaches and the resulting decreased resolution, small thrombi within the anterosuperior and lateral left atrium are difficult to identify using TTE. In addition, it has been shown that TEE-detected spontaneous echo contrast of the left atrium is an indicator for increased thromboembolic events in patients with mitral stenosis or a mitral prosthesis.[9]

DISEASES OF THE THORACIC AORTA

TEE is a superb technique for the evaluation of aortic dissections and is emerging as the procedure of choice for the diagnosis and follow-up of this condition (see Ch. 9). Erbel et al.[10] described a sensitivity and specificity for diagnosing aortic dissection of 97 percent and 100 percent, respectively. Biplane TEE is the ideal initial screening test because of its ability to visualize the whole thoracic aorta. TEE is capable of showing the morphology and extent of the dissection and the entrance and exit of the false lumen and can be used to evaluate the results of treatment without exposing a dangerously ill patient to the risk of transportation to other imaging facilities.

Using TEE, recurrent peripheral arterial embolization was shown to be due to protruding atheroma with friable material or thrombus in the descending aorta, probably originating from advanced-stage arteriosclerosis in the aorta.[11]

COMPLICATIONS OF MYOCARDIAL INFARCTION

TEE is useful in the evaluation of mechanical complications following acute myocardial infarction, such as ventricular septal rupture, papillary muscle rupture, papillary muscle dysfunction (Fig. 15-1), and pseudoaneurysm (see Ch. 13). Another useful application of TEE is the evaluation of right ventricular function in the setting of right ventricular infarction and cardiogenic shock (Fig. 15-2).

CARDIAC TAMPONADE

Two-dimensional TTE is the study of choice for the diagnosis of pericardial effusion and cardiac tam-

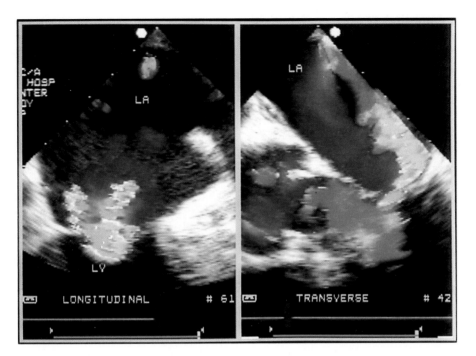

Fig. 15-1. Biplane imaging of mitral regurgitation in a patient with an inferoposterior myocardial infarction and posteromedial papillary muscle dysfunction. There is moderate mitral regurgitation. LA, left atrium; LV, left ventricle.

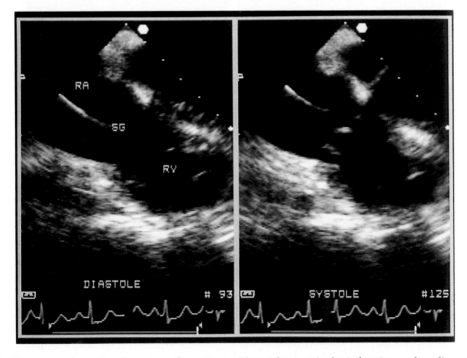

Fig. 15-2. Transverse four-chamber view of a patient with a right ventricular infarction and cardiogenic shock. The right ventricle (RV) is dilated, and there is marked impairment in contractility during systole. RA, right atrium; SG, Swan-Ganz catheter.

ponade. Early and late diastolic collapse of the right ventricle and right atrium by 2-D TTE has been found to be a fairly reliable sign of hemodynamically compromised cardiac tamponade.[12] Right atrial inversion is more sensitive than right ventricular collapse.

In patients with tamponade, Doppler echocardiography shows a marked inspiratory increase (more than 40 percent) in tricuspid and pulmonary flow velocity and an exaggerated decrease (more than 40 percent) in mitral and aortic velocity.[12] Such velocity "paradoxus" also can occur in patients with obstructive lung disease.

Cardiac tamponade can have unusual features and presents in an atypical fashion, particularly after cardiac surgery.[13] A loculated hematoma can often be difficult to detect with conventional TTE in these patients because of poor image quality. Surgical wounds and dressings, mechanical ventilators and intraaortic balloon pump limit the ability to obtain high-quality echocardiograms. TEE has been found to be superior to TTE in evaluating critically ill postoperative hypotensive patients in whom a loculated pericardial hematoma has developed after cardiac surgery with clinical findings of tamponade.[14] In the four cases reported, a large hematoma was found to be compressing the entire anterior surface of the right atrium.[14]

We have performed TEE studies in postoperative cardiac surgical patients in whom hypotension has developed after surgery. TEE is useful in the postoperative hypotensive patient and can differentiate cardiac tamponade or isolated right atrial tamponade from other causes of hemodynamic deterioration, such as prosthetic valve dysfunction or left ventricular systolic dysfunction, or both (Fig. 15-3).

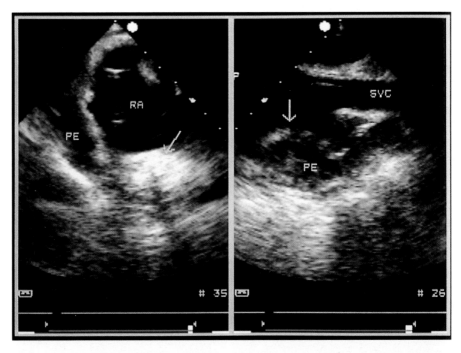

Fig. 15-3. Biplane view of the right atrium in a patient who developed hypotension after coronary artery bypass surgery. *(Left)* Transverse plane demonstrating a large loculated hematoma (arrow) and pericardial effusion (PE) anterior to the right atrium (RA). *(Right)* Longitudinal plane at level of superior vena cava (SVC) showing right atrial wall inversion (arrow) and pericardial effusion (PE). Surgical exploration revealed a loculated hematoma compressing the anterior surface of the right atrium.

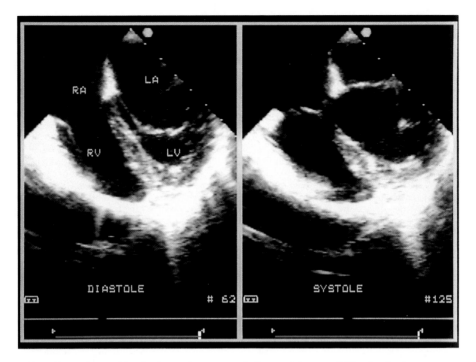

Fig. 15-4. TEE study performed in the intensive care unit from a 21-year-old brain-dead woman considered a potential cardiac donor. Transverse four-chamber views in diastole and systole. The complete study was normal. The transthoracic study was technically suboptimal and nondiagnostic. LA, left atrium; LV, left ventricle; RA, right atrium; RV, right ventricle.

TRAUMATIC HEART DISEASE

Penetrating and nonpenetrating chest trauma can damage the myocardium, pericardium, cardiac valves, and great vessels. In a case of penetrating chest injury, the patient may require immediate surgery, precluding an echocardiographic study. TTE is limited in these patients because of life-support devices and the inability to position the patient properly for a standard transthoracic study. Furthermore, TTE is limited in visualizing the entire thoracic aorta and in the evaluation of right ventricular function.

TEE can be performed in the emergency department, and excellent images of intracardiac structures and great vessels can be obtained. TEE can determine the presence or absence of hemopericardium and tamponade, as well as a laceration or tear of the myocardium, great vessels, ventricular and atrial septa, and valves. Should immediate surgery be warranted, either intraoperative or early postoperative TEE may be useful to rule out associated intracardiac damage.

EVALUATING POTENTIAL DONOR HEARTS

TEE is useful in evaluating potential donor hearts for cardiac transplantation (Fig. 15-4). Cardiac tamponade, myocardial contusion, and laceration or tear of the myocardium, great vessels, and valvular damage can be rapidly assessed by TEE. This information can be acquired quite rapidly, and decisions can be made as to the appropriateness of harvesting the donor heart.

REFERENCES

1. Oh JK, Seward JB, Khandheria BK. Transesophageal echocardiography in the intensive care unit. Circulation 1988; 78(suppl II):298 (abst).
2. Patel AM, Miller FA, Khandheria BK, et al. Role of transesophageal echocardiography in the diagnosis of papillary muscle rupture secondary to myocardial infarction. Am Heart J 1989; 118:1330–1335.
3. Font VE, Obarski TP, Klein AL, et al. Transesophageal echocardiography in the critical care unit. Cleve Clin J Med 1991; 58:315–322.

4. Mills TJ, Talierco CP, Bailey KR, et al. Transthoracic versus transesophageal two-dimensional echo/Doppler flow imaging in surgical patients with mitral regurgitation. J Am Coll Cardiol 1989; 13:68A (abst).

5. Nellessen U, Schnittger I, Appleton CP, et al. Transesophageal two-dimensional echocardiography and color Doppler flow velocity mapping in the evaluation of cardiac valve prostheses. Circulation 1988; 78:848–855.

6. Currie PJ, Calafiore P, Stewart WJ, et al. Transesophageal echo in mitral prosthetic dysfunction: echo-surgical correlation. J Am Coll Cardiol 1989; 13:69A (abst).

7. Khandheria B, Seward J, Oh J, et al. Mitral prosthesis malfunction: utility of transesophageal echocardiography. J Am Coll Cardiol 1989; 13:69A (abst).

8. Mügge A, Daniel WG, Frank G, et al. Echocardiography in infective endocarditis: reassessment of prognostic implications of vegetation size determined by the transthoracic and the transesophageal approach. J Am Coll Cardiol 1989; 14:631–638.

9. Daniel WG, Nellessen U, Schroder E, et al. Left atrial spontaneous echo contrast in mitral valve disease: an indicator for an increased thromboembolic risk. J Am Coll Cardiol 1988; 11:1204–1211.

10. Erbel R, Mohr-Kahaly S, Rennollet H, et al. Diagnosis of aortic dissection: the value of transesophageal echocardiography. Thorac Cardiovasc Surg 1987; 35:126–133.

11. Tunick PA, Kronzon I. Protruding atherosclerotic plaque in the aortic arch of patients with systemic embolization: a new finding seen by transesophageal echocardiography. Am Heart J 1990; 120:658–662.

12. Pandian NG, Weintraub A, Kusay BS, et al. Emergency echocardiography. Echocardiography 1989; 6:45–61.

13. Shabetai R. Changing concepts of cardiac tamponade. (Editorial.) J Am Coll Cardiol 1988; 12:194–195.

14. Kochar GS, Jacobs LE, Kotler MN. Right atrial compression in postoperative cardiac patients: detection by transesophageal echocardiography. J Am Coll Cardiol 1990; 16:511–516.

16 Intraoperative Applications

Intraoperative TEE has proved particularly valuable in patients undergoing either cardiac or noncardiac surgery. The intraoperative uses of this approach can be divided into three major categories: monitoring of cardiac function, detailed intraoperative diagnosis, and detection of intracardiac air embolism. (For specific indications for intraoperative TEE, see Ch. 3, Table 3-1.)

This chapter reviews the use of intraoperative echocardiography in patients undergoing mitral and tricuspid valve repair, aortic valve surgery and relief of left ventricular outflow tract obstruction, and detection of retained intracardiac air. (For a review of intraoperative monitoring of ischemia and cardiac function, see Ch. 17.)

INTRAOPERATIVE ASSESSMENT OF VALVE REPAIR

Intraoperative assessment of the competence of reconstructed atrioventricular valves is an important application of TEE. Repair procedures that preserve a patient's native valve offer a number of advantages over prosthetic valve replacement. Mitral valvuloplasty is associated with significantly fewer valve-related complications than occur with prosthetic replacement, including a lower perioperative and a 7-year mortality and a lower incidence of thromboembolic events.[3] Preservation of left ventricular function is also better with mitral valve repair than with prosthetic replacement,[4,5] presumably because the continuity between left ventricular wall, mitral apparatus, and mitral annulus is not disrupted.[6] Tricuspid valve repair is also being performed with increasing frequency, since uncorrected severe tricuspid regurgitation has been shown to result in substantial postoperative morbidity, and even mortality.[7]

Mitral valve repair operations have been performed in relatively few centers in the past because regurgitation frequently persists after repair[8,9] and because the adequacy of repair can be difficult to evaluate at surgery.[10] Although mild residual regurgitation may be considered acceptable, more severe regurgitation can lead to hemodynamic complications and may require subsequent reoperation. Intraoperative assessment of the success of valve repair surgery using conventional methods has been fraught with some difficulties and has contributed to the reluctance to perform reconstructive valve surgery. TEE provides high-quality real-time tomographic images of cardiac morphologic characteristics and intracardiac blood flow and is thus uniquely suited to provide intraoperative information about the adequacy of valve repair procedures.

Conventional Assessment of Valve Repair

Traditionally employed procedures for intraoperative assessment of the adequacy of repair offer only limited information[10-13] and are often poor predictors of outcome. Fluid injection into the arrested ventricle for assessment of valve leakage has been used widely.[14,15] With this approach, however, both the geometry and chamber pressure of the nonbeating heart are different from the physiologic state. This

157

Table 16-1. Echocardiography in Valve Repair

Timing	Imaging Modality	Purpose
Preoperative	TTE,[a] TEE	Identify candidates for, and timing of, surgery
		Determine mechanism and severity of regurgitation and feasibility of repair
Intraoperative Prepump	TEE,[b] EE	Assess ventricular function
		Refine understanding of mechanism
		Obtain baseline information
Postpump		Identify failed repairs
		Determine mechanism of persistent regurgitation
		Identify surgical complications
		Detect air embolism
Postoperative	TTE,[a] TEE	Document successful repair
		Compare preoperative and postoperative ventricular function
		Identify late failed repairs
		Follow patient serially

Abbreviations: EE, epicardial echo; TEE, transesophageal echocardiography; TTE, transthoracic echocardiography.
[a] Preferred for initial baseline study.
[b] Procedure of choice.

can lead to both underestimation as well as overestimation of the degree of regurgitation that will occur subsequently in the beating heart. Measurement of atrial pressure and the height of V-waves may also be misleading, since they are very dependent on atrial size and compliance, as well as on preload and afterload conditions.[12–13,16] Palpating the atria for the presence of systolic thrills also has not proved a reliable approach in the intraoperative evaluation of mitral and tricuspid regurgitation.

Imaging Methodology

Echocardiography is indicated at four points in the management of patients undergoing repair of regurgitant mitral and tricuspid valves: preoperatively, in the operating room before and after cardiopulmonary bypass, and postoperatively. The intraoperative study can be performed using either an epicardial or a transesophageal approach (Table 16-1).

For epicardial imaging, a 3.5- or 5.0-MHz transducer is covered with a sterile plastic sleeve and placed directly on the surface of the heart. Ultrasonic coupling gel is placed between the transducer surface and the inside of the sleeve; to improve the acoustic interface between the outer surface of the sleeve and the epicardium, the latter is moistened with sterile saline solution. From this point, the mitral valve can be imaged in multiple long-axis and short-axis planes. By moving the transducer assembly inferiorly toward the diaphragmatic surface of the right ventricle, the tricuspid valve can be imaged in subxiphoid equivalent long-axis and short-axis views. Epicardial views may be difficult to obtain in reoperated patients with adhesive pericarditis and in patients with excessive epicardial fat.[17]

Intraoperative TEE imaging is performed as previously described in Chapter 3. Imaging is performed before cardiopulmonary bypass. Simultaneously, right atrial, pulmonary arterial, and systemic arterial pressures are recorded from pulmonary and arterial catheters. A second intraoperative TEE study is performed after cardiopulmonary bypass and rewarming, but before decannulation.

Transesophageal Versus Epicardial Echocardiography

Transesophageal imaging has several advantages over epicardial imaging (Table 16-2). It can be initi-

Table 16-2. Comparison of Epicardial vs. Transesophageal Echocardiography

Advantages	Disadvantages
Epicardial Imaging	
1. High-quality images	1. Interrupts sterile surgical field
2. Multiple tomographic planes	2. Poor visualization of apex of left ventricle
3. Continuous-wave Doppler capability	3. Arrhythmias, if press too firmly
	4. Learning curve to image moving heart
	5. Assessment of mitral prosthetic regurgitation difficult
Transesophageal Imaging	
1. Biplane probe permits transverse and longitudinal imaging planes	1. Single-plane probe: fewer tomographic imaging planes
2. No interruption of surgical field	2. Difficult to insert probe once anesthetic shield in place
3. Continuous monitoring during surgery	3. Artifacts from electrocautery
4. Continuous-wave Doppler available in newer probes	4. Monopolizes the TEE probe for entire operation
5. Optimal for assessment of mitral prosthetic regurgitation	

ated immediately after the induction of general anesthesia and adds no time to the length of the surgical procedure. In addition, imaging can be performed continuously without interfering with the operation. This approach makes on-line data available to the surgeon and the anesthesiologist regarding left ventricular function, regional wall-motion abnormalities, valvular function, and the presence of intracardiac air. It offers excellent images of a number of structures, including the left atrium, mitral valve, and descending thoracic aorta. Prosthetic valves in the mitral or aortic position do not interfere with imaging of left atrial structures and mitral regurgitant jets.

The image planes obtainable by conventional single-plane TEE may be limited, since the ability to position the transducer is restricted by the confines of the esophagus. This can be an important limitation when evaluating complex congenital heart disease. Even in acquired heart disease, some structures can be difficult to visualize at times, such as the tricuspid valve in the presence of a calcified and dilated aorta.

Biplane TEE, which has recently become widely available, overcomes many of these limitations. The addition of a longitudinal image plane allows for a more complete and detailed evaluation of cardiac structures and of the great vessels. Even with this technique, however, the left ventricle can be difficult to image from behind the left atrium in the presence of a mitral prosthesis, but it may be visualized in transgastric views. The newer transesophageal probes have continuous-wave Doppler capability. Its clinical value includes measurement of mitral stenotic gradients and estimation of right ventricular systolic pressures from tricuspid regurgitant velocities. Aortic valve gradients can often be measured using a transgastric approach. However, they are generally not used in the standard transesophageal views designed to image the aortic valve, since flow in these views is nearly perpendicular to the interrogating beam.

The major advantages of intraoperative epicardial echocardiography include the ability (1) to obtain high-quality images quickly from multiple tomographic planes; and (2) to estimate the pressure gradient across the left ventricular outflow tract, using the nonimaging continuous-wave Doppler transducer on the ascending aorta.

A major limitation of the epicardial technique is poor visualization of the apex of the left ventricle. Similarly, an accurate mitral valve gradient cannot be obtained by continuous-wave Doppler epicardial echocardiography because it fails to align the beam parallel to flow. In addition, epicardial echocardiography interrupts the operation and enters the surgical field. If the echocardiographer presses too firmly on the heart with the epicardial transducer, arrhythmias may occur. Image quality may deteriorate when there is diffuse epicardial scarring, as occurs in patients who have adhesions from previous operations, in those who have had pericarditis, and in those with excessive epicardial fat. Large hearts can be difficult to scan, particularly when much of the heart lies underneath the chest wall, even when the latter is maximally retracted.

Physiologic Considerations

Careful attention must be paid to factors that can greatly affect regurgitant severity, including ventricular afterload, preload, inotropic state, and myocardial temperature.

Atrioventricular valve regurgitation is particularly sensitive to the afterload state. In the operating room, the patient's afterload is often markedly affected by anesthesia and by commonly administered pharmacologic agents. Careful consideration should therefore be given to the patient's peripheral systolic blood pressure when one is evaluating mitral regurgitation[11,12] and to pulmonary arterial systolic pressure when one is evaluating tricuspid regurgitation.[13] For this reason, we routinely administer intravenous phenylephrine when these pressures are below the preoperative levels to increase systolic pressure to a level that is comparable to the patient's ambulatory pressure. At the very least, we try to raise systemic systolic pressure to a level of 120 to 140 mmHg. The increase in color Doppler regurgitant area is highly variable among individual patients, ranging from very mild to very severe (Fig. 16-1).

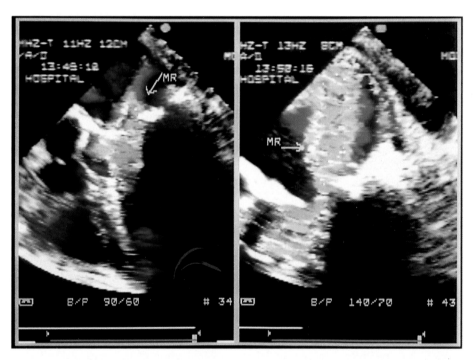

Fig. 16-1. Postcardiopulmonary bypass study following mitral valve repair with a Carpentier-Edwards ring. *(Left)* Mild mitral regurgitation (MR) at a blood pressure below preoperative level. *(Right)* An increase in systolic pressure after administration of intravenous phenylephrine was associated with a significant increase in mitral regurgitation (MR), indicating unsatisfactory operative results. The patient subsequently underwent mitral valve replacement.

The preload state is also an important factor, and we therefore try to pay attention to the patient's volume status. Particularly in the setting after cardiopulmonary bypass, during evaluation of the adequacy of valve repair, the patient should be transfused and should have received an appropriate amount of intravenous fluids. The pulmonary capillary wedge pressure can serve as a useful guideline in this setting. Importantly, final evaluation of valvular regurgitation should not take place too early after completion of cardiopulmonary bypass, since at that time myocardial function can still be greatly affected by cardioplegia and hypothermia. Nevertheless, since cardiac function and hemodynamics can be quite variable at this time, continuous monitoring of valvular regurgitation and ventricular function may be required until chest closure, or even until the stabilization of hemodynamics in the intensive care unit.

The ability to do so constitutes an additional advantage of the transesophageal approach as an intraoperative monitoring tool.

Precardiopulmonary Bypass

Annular and Atrial Size

With chronic regurgitation, the atrium and the annulus dilate, and the annulus loses its elliptical shape, becoming more circular. Annular dilation in turn leads to poor coaptation of the valve leaflets and worsening of incompetence (Fig. 16-2). Reestablishment of a normal annular size and shape can reduce or eliminate regurgitation in this setting (Figs. 16-3 and 16-4). Thus, an annulus-reducing procedure is nearly always required when annular dilation is present. In acute regurgitation, atrial and annular size

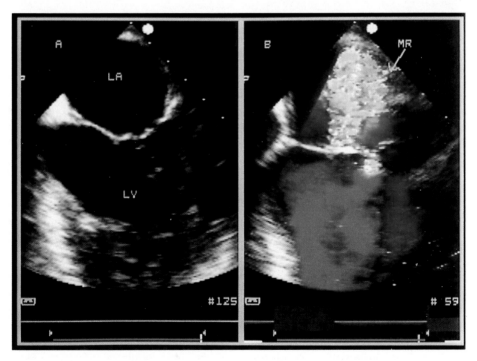

Fig. 16-2. *(Left)* Transverse midesophageal view of patient with annular dilatation and dilated left atrium (LA). *(Right)* Color Doppler showing severe mitral regurgitation (MR). LV, left ventricle.

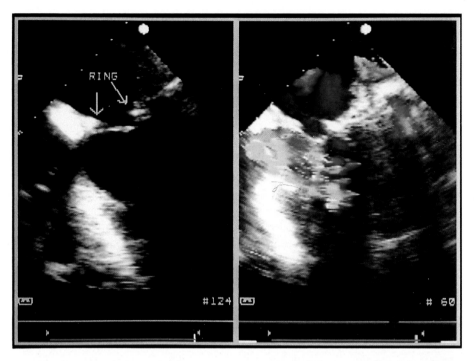

Fig. 16-3. Postoperative study of same patient shown in Figure 16-2. *(Left)* Reestablishment of normal annular size with a Carpentier-Edwards ring. *(Right)* Color Doppler image showing no mitral regurgitation.

are usually normal, and an annulus-reducing procedure is often not required. Rather, other techniques of repair are indicated. The need for an annulus-reducing procedure can therefore be determined by echocardiographic measurement of atrial and annular size.

Leaflets and Chordae

Myxomatous degeneration may produce ballooning and scalloping of the valve leaflets; this valvular redundancy can be identified echocardiographically (Figs. 16-5 and 16-6). Myxomatous degeneration may also produce localized areas of thinning and thickening that can be seen echocardiographically. Marked prolapse or leaflet malalignment may be present, resulting from chordal elongation. Ruptured chords are identified by their appearance in the atrium during systole (Figs. 16-7 and 16-8). In patients with active endocarditis, vegetations may be attached to the leaflets or chords. With rheumatic valve disease, thickening and/or calcification of the leaflets, restriction of leaflet motion, and a variable degree of shortening and thickening of the subvalvular apparatus may be identified (Fig. 16-9). In patients experiencing regurgitation caused by coronary artery disease, the leaflets and chords appear normal. Thus, pathologic changes in the leaflets and/or chords and the etiologic basis of the regurgitation can be determined by TEE. This information aids in planning the surgical procedure.

Papillary Muscles and Wall Motion

Segmental wall-motion abnormalities are a hallmark of coronary artery disease and may be produced by reversible ischemia or infarction (Fig. 16-10). Thinning of the myocardium, atresia of the papillary muscles, and dyskinetic wall segments are indicative of prior remote infarction. These findings may be helpful in establishing the etiologic basis of regurgitation

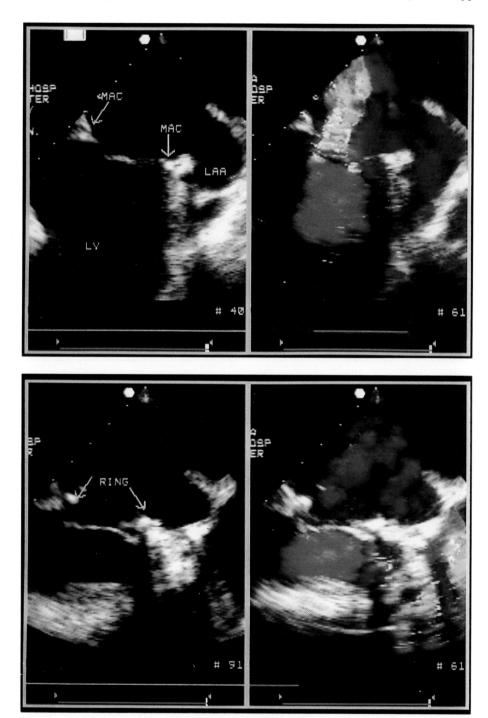

Fig. 16-4. *(Top left)* Longitudinal two-chamber view demonstrating mitral annular calcification (MAC). *(Top right)* Color Doppler showing moderate mitral regurgitation. *(Bottom left)* Postoperative study following repair with a Carpentier-Edwards ring and coronary artery bypass grafting. *(Bottom right)* Color Doppler showing no evidence of residual mitral regurgitation. LAA, left atrial appendage; LV, left ventricle.

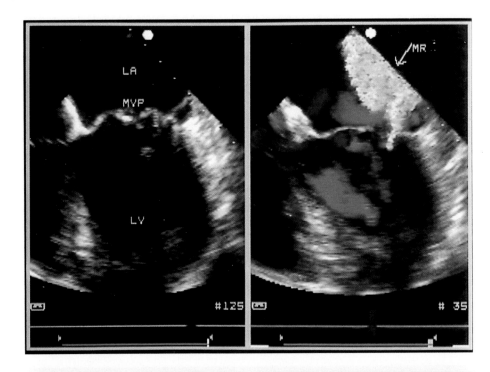

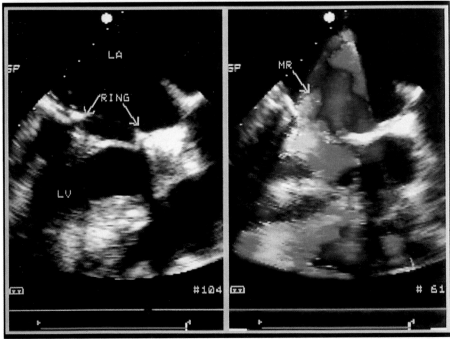

Fig. 16-5. *(Top left)* Transverse two-chamber view demonstrating mitral valve prolapse (MVP) involving both anterior and posterior leaflets. The valve is thickened and redundant. *(Top right)* Color Doppler showing moderate mitral regurgitation (MR). *(Bottom left)* Longitudinal view after mitral valve repair with a Duran annuplasty ring, quadrangular resection of the posterior leaflet, and chordal transfer to the anterior mitral leaflet. *(Bottom right)* Color Doppler showing mild residual mitral regurgitation (MR). LA, left atrium; LV, left ventricle.

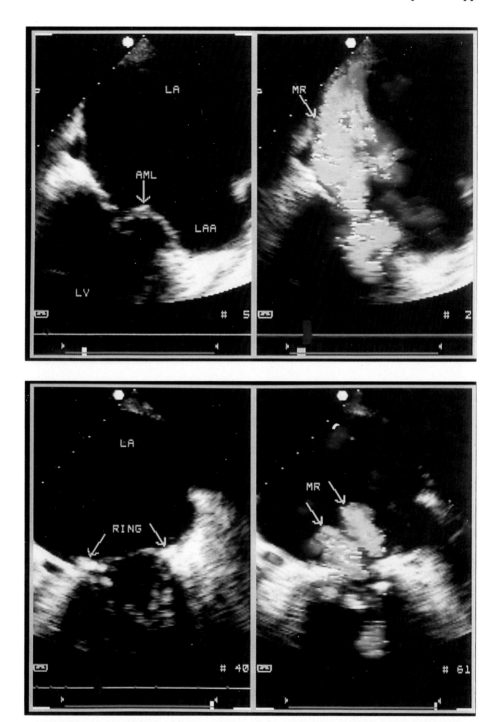

Fig. 16-6. Longitudinal two-chamber view. *(Top left)* Prolapse of the anterior mitral leaflet (AML). Note the thickened, redundant valve. *(Top right)* Color Doppler showing moderate-severe mitral regurgitation (MR). *(Bottom left)* Mitral valve repair with a Duran ring and chordal transfer to the anterior leaflet. *(Bottom right)* Color Doppler showing mild residual mitral regurgitation (MR). LA, left atrium; LAA, left atrial appendage; LV, left ventricle.

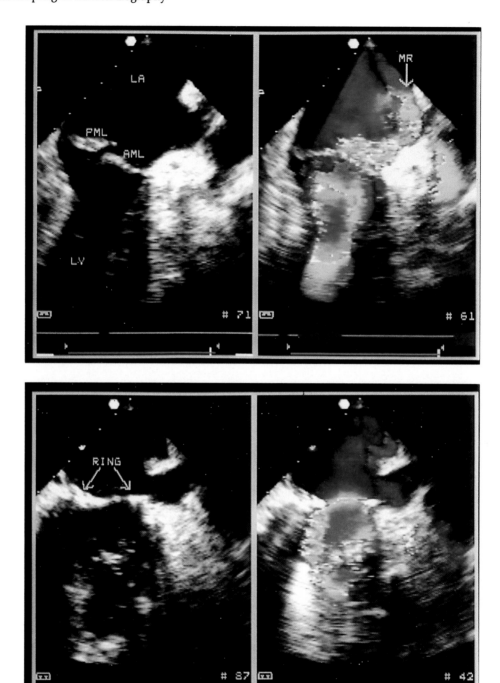

Fig. 16-7. *(Top left)* Preoperative longitudinal two-chamber view demonstrating a flail posterior mitral leaflet due to ruptured chordae tendineae. *(Top right)* Color Doppler image showing significant mitral regurgitation (MR). The eccentric regurgitant jet is directed anteriorly. *(Bottom left)* Mitral valve repair with a Carpentier-Edwards ring and quadrangular resection of the posterior leaflet. *(Bottom right)* Color Doppler image showing no mitral regurgitation. AML, anterior mitral leaflet; LA, left atrium; LV, left ventricle.

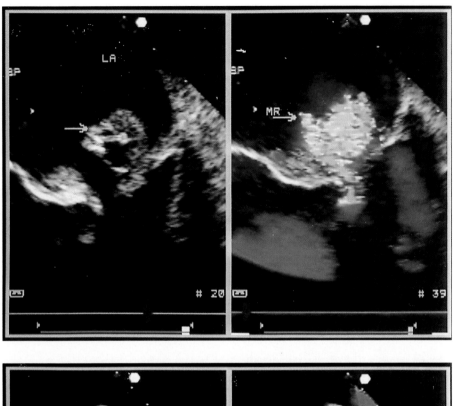

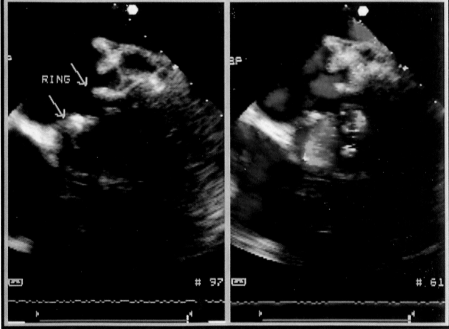

Fig. 16-8. Transverse two-chamber view. *(Top left)* Preoperative study showing a flail posterior mitral leaflet (arrow). *(Top right)* Color Doppler demonstrating significant mitral regurgitation (MR). *(Bottom left)* Postoperative study after mitral valve repair with a Duran ring and resection of posterior mitral leaflet. *(Bottom right)* Color Doppler showing no mitral regurgitation. LA, left atrium.

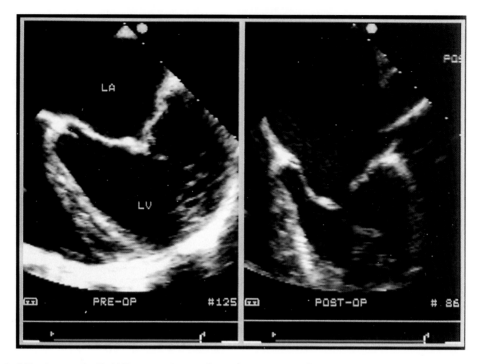

Fig. 16-9. Mitral stenosis. *(Left)* Preoperative study in the transverse four-chamber view at end-diastole, showing doming of the mitral valve along with thickening. *(Right)* Postoperative study after open commissurotomy. There is marked improvement in valve area determined by spectral Doppler. LA, left atrium; LV, left ventricle.

caused by coronary artery disease. Atretic papillary muscles can be identified by their diminutive size and increased echocardiographic density on short-axis imaging (Fig. 16-11).

Direction of Regurgitant Jet

Jet direction may provide corroborative evidence of leaflet prolapse and chordal elongation. For example, in a patient with mitral regurgitation, a jet directed under the anterior mitral leaflet is associated with prolapse of the posterior leaflet. Similarly, a jet directed along the inferior or free posterolateral wall of the left atrium is associated with anterior leaflet prolapse.

Origin of the Regurgitant Jet

In patients with regurgitation caused by ischemic heart disease, the origin of the jet in relationship to the commissure may be helpful in guiding surgical decision making. The mitral commissure may be divided arbitrarily into thirds: the inferior portion (adjacent to the inferior wall of the left ventricle), the middle portion, and the superior portion (adjacent to the anterolateral wall of the left ventricle). The mitral commissure and the origin of the jet can be imaged from the transesophageal approach by reflecting the transducer upward after passing through the gastroesophageal junction into the stomach. Ischemic mitral regurgitation originates from the inferior commissure or from the central portion of the commissure in nearly all patients.[18]

Importantly, the origin of the jet correlates with the success of valve repair by a suture annuloplasty technique. Jets originating from the inferior commissure are best treated by a suture annuloplasty, with a 90 percent success rate, whereas central jets usually require a ring annuloplasty.

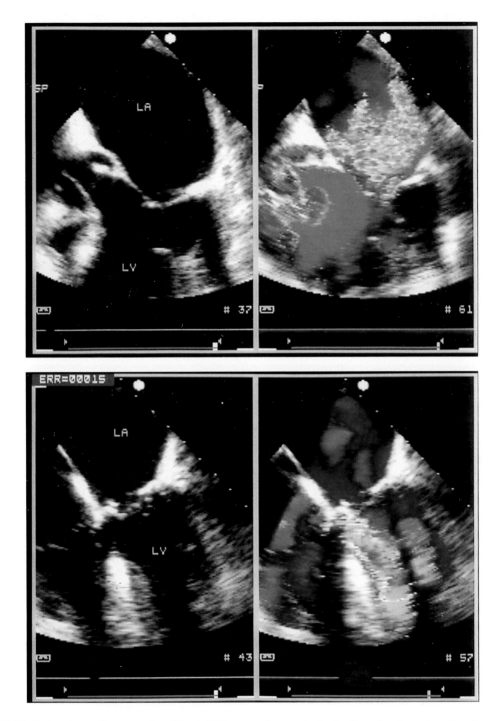

Fig. 16-10. Ischemic cardiomyopathy. *(Top left)* Preoperative study in the five-chamber view showing a morphologic normal mitral valve. The left atrium (LA) and left ventricle (LV) are dilated. *(Top right)* Color Doppler image showing severe mitral regurgitation. *(Bottom left)* After coronary artery bypass and placement of annuloplasty ring. *(Bottom right)* Color Doppler showing no residual mitral regurgitation.

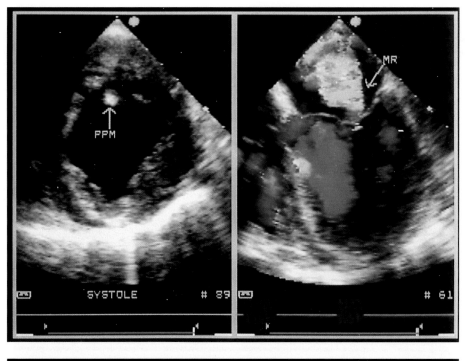

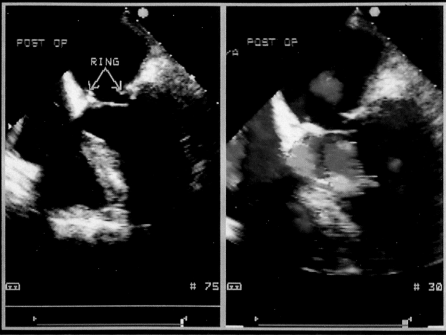

Fig. 16-11. Papillary muscle dysfunction. *(Top left)* Transgastric short-axis view at end-systole showing akinesis of the posterior wall and scarring of the posteromedial papillary muscle (PPM). Note the increased echo density of the PPM. *(Top right)* Color Doppler in the transverse four-chamber view showing severe mitral regurgitation (MR). *(Bottom left)* Postoperative study after mitral valve repair with a Duran ring. *(Bottom right)* No residual mitral regurgitation on color Doppler.

VALVE REPAIR PROCEDURES

Myxomatous degeneration of the valve with localized scalloping of the posterior leaflet or ruptured chordae is ideally suited for repair. The most common operation is resection of a prolapsed posterior leaflet (that may or may not have ruptured chordae), closure of the resected margins, and placement of an annuloplasty ring. Several types of prosthetic rings are available, including the Carpentier-Edwards, Duran, and Puig-Massana rings. Complications of annuloplasty include stenosis (from overcorrection) and outflow tract obstruction (from rigid mitral rings, such as the Carpentier-Edwards).[19]

In ischemic mitral regurgitation, an annuloplasty ring may be all that is needed. In the patient with ischemic mitral regurgitation who has ruptured chordae, localized resection should suffice.

Multiple elongated chordae can be repaired by various shortening procedures; redundant leaflet tissue is removed by triangular wedge resection or quadrilateral resection and reapproximation of the leaflet edges. Clefts are closed by direct suture repair. Holes on the leaflet are patched with pericardial tissue. Calcific deposits are debrided by careful curettage.

Repair of the anterior leaflet, alone or in combination with the posterior leaflet, is more difficult. Repair of the anterior leaflet with chordal rupture or elongation requires attachment of the ruptured chordae to an adjacent large chord. Alternatively, a chordal transfer of a segment of posterior leaflet to the anterior leaflet may be performed.

In patients with rheumatic mitral regurgitation, commissurotomy, debriding of the calcified valve leaflets, resection of portions of leaflets, and remodeling with annuloplasty may be necessary. In those with endocarditis, with a simple perforation in a valve leaflet or localized ruptured chordae, resection is used, or small pieces of pericardium may be inserted as a patch to bridge the defect. In the event of annular disruption, valve replacement and more involved procedures to repair the annulus with pericardial patch material may be required.

Postcardiopulmonary Bypass

Once the patient has come off bypass, intraoperative TEE evaluates the presence, severity, and the mechanism of residual regurgitation after valve repair for regurgitant lesions.[20] Defining the mechanism of the residual regurgitation is important in the surgical decision-making process. When immediate reoperation is required in the patient with a failed mitral repair, the surgeon must have an immediate optimal understanding of the mechanism of the failed repair (e.g., suture line dehiscence, dynamic left ventricular outflow obstruction, or residual mitral regurgitation from incomplete repair) in order to make an informed decision as to whether the valve should be re-repaired or replaced.[21,22] For those patients who have undergone valve repair for stenosis, intraoperative TEE can assess new or increased valvular regurgitation (e.g., after open mitral commissurotomy). In addition, steerable continuous-wave Doppler velocity measurements can be made, and the valve area can be calculated from the pressure half-time of transvalvular diastolic flow. In general, the orifice area should be greater than $1.0 \text{ cm}^2/\text{m}^2$ of body surface area. Overcorrection of regurgitation by insertion of a small ring can produce functional stenosis.

Left ventricular outflow tract obstruction is a well-described complication that occurs in 4.5 percent to 6 percent of patients undergoing mitral annuloplasty with a rigid Carpentier-Edwards ring.[23,24] This finding is associated with systolic anterior motion of the mitral leaflets without prior evidence of asymmetric septal hypertrophy (Figs. 16-12 to 16-14). Left ventricular outflow tract obstruction has not been described after suture annuloplasty or annuloplasty using the flexible Duran ring.

We have observed an unusual complication following mitral annuloplasty with a rigid Carpentier-Edwards ring. TEE demonstrated new-onset severe aortic regurgitation caused by an inadvertent suture of an aortic valve cusp producing incomplete coaptation of the aortic valve (Fig. 16-15). Cardiopulmonary bypass was reinstituted and corrective action taken.

In patients who are not candidates for valve repair and who receive a prosthetic valve, intraoperative TEE can accurately detect prosthetic dysfunction,[25] especially periprosthetic regurgitation (e.g., after su-

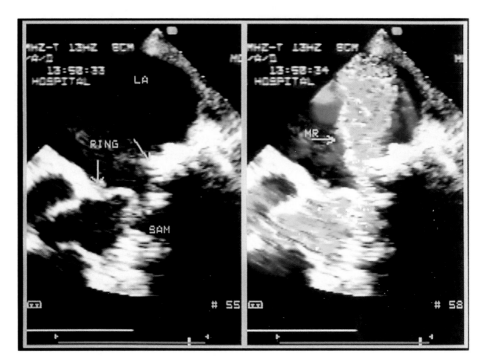

Fig. 16-12. Failed mitral valve repair. *(Left)* Transverse midesophageal view demonstrating a rigid Carpentier-Edwards ring and systolic anterior motion (SAM) of the mitral valve producing obstruction to left ventricular outflow. *(Right)* Color Doppler showing severe mitral regurgitation (MR) and turbulent flow in the left ventricular outflow tract caused by obstruction. LA, left atrium.

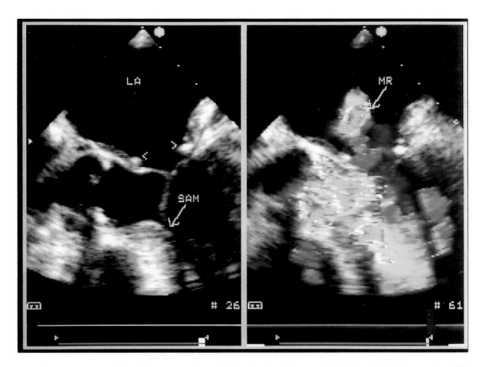

Fig. 16-13. *(Left)* Transverse plane from a patient with mitral valve repair with a rigid Carpentier-Edwards ring (arrowheads) and systolic anterior motion (SAM) of the mitral leaflets producing left ventricular outflow obstruction. *(Right)* Color Doppler image showing mild residual mitral regurgitation (MR) and a mosaic color pattern in the left ventricular outflow tract caused by obstruction. LA, left atrium.

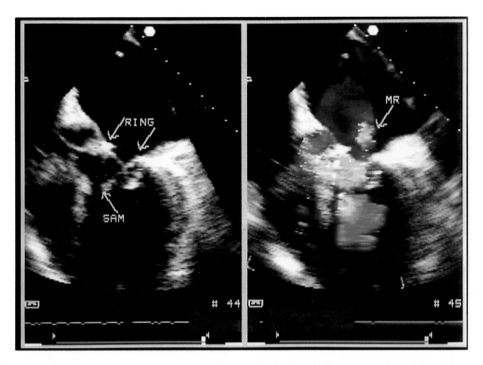

Fig. 16-14. *(Left)* Systolic anterior motion (SAM) of the mitral valve following repair with a rigid Carpentier-Edwards ring. *(Right)* Color Doppler showing minimal mitral regurgitation (MR). No corrective action was taken, and the patient remains asymptomatic.

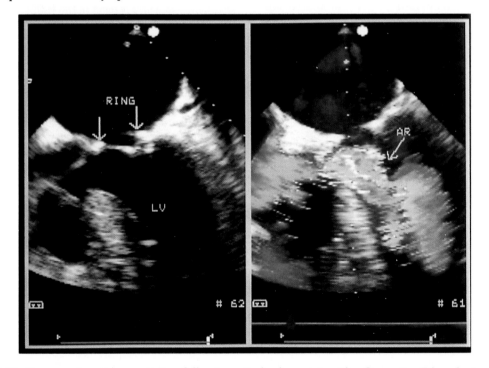

Fig. 16-15. New-onset aortic regurgitation following mitral valve repair with a Carpentier-Edwards ring. *(Left)* Transverse five-chamber view demonstrating the mitral ring. *(Right)* Color Doppler showing severe aortic regurgitation (AR). LV, left ventricle.

ture closure of a periprosthetic leak, or prosthetic valve replacement).[26]

Follow-up of Valve Repair

We generally obtain a transthoracic echocardiogram (TTE) before discharging the patient, or within the first 2 months after surgery. The purpose is to document that the repair was successful, to assess early postrepair left ventricular function, to determine the degree of improvement in pulmonary hypertension, and to provide a baseline under ambulatory conditions for serial postoperative comparisons.

Late postoperative failure of mitral valvuloplasty requiring reoperation varies from 1 percent to 3.9 percent and is higher during the first year after surgery, when technical failures or unrecognized additional lesions become manifest.[27] From 2 to 10 years postoperatively, the most common cause of valve repair failure is the recurrence or progression of disease.[28] Less common causes of reoperation are endocarditis, hemolysis, and iatrogenic stenosis. The presence of mild mitral regurgitation detected by clinical examination or Doppler echocardiography does not predict the need for late reoperation.[9] Left ventricular outflow obstruction is usually detected by intraoperative echocardiography and can be corrected immediately with valve replacement or by removal of the annuloplasty ring.

Chordal rupture as a late complication after mitral valve reconstruction was reported in three cases of chordal rupture at an interval after mitral valve reconstruction involving chordal shortening procedures.[29] Each patient had severe recurrent mitral regurgitation requiring reoperation and mitral valve replacement. This problem of late chordal rupture after repair of the mitral valve for myxomatous degeneration appears to be an infrequent but definite complication of current chordal shortening techniques.

SURGICAL REPAIR OF THE AORTIC VALVE AND LEFT VENTRICULAR OUTFLOW TRACT OBSTRUCTION

The introduction of the biplane TEE probe permits much greater ease in obtaining orthogonal imaging of the aortic valve and left ventricular outflow tract.

Table 16-3. Indications for Intraoperative Echocardiographic Evaluation of the Aortic Valve and Left Ventricular Outflow Tract

Aortic valve repair
    Aortic stenosis
    Aortic regurgitation
Aortic homograft
Complications following aortic valve replacement
Septal myectomy for hypertrophic obstructive cardiomyopathy
Discrete membranous or muscular tunnel subaortic stenosis

The incorporation of continuous-wave Doppler to the esophageal probe makes it feasible to quantify the severity of left ventricular outflow tract obstruction both before and after cardiopulmonary bypass (Table 16-3).

Aortic Stenosis

Aortic valve replacement is the procedure of choice for most patients who have symptomatic severe valvular aortic stenosis. Intraoperative echocardiography is probably unnecessary in most patients undergoing aortic valve replacement. Intraoperative echocardiography is used in the following situations:

1. Preoperative evaluation suggests the feasibility of aortic valve repair.
2. Associated mitral valve pathology is present.
3. Difficulty is encountered in separating the patient from cardiopulmonary bypass[30]
4. In cases with concomitant subvalvular obstruction.[31-32]
5. In patients undergoing a second aortic valve replacement in whom periprosthetic regurgitation was present and the surgeon attempted suture closure of the perivalvular leak.[33]

There has recently been a resurgence of interest in the surgical repair of calcific stenotic aortic valves. Surgical valvuloplasty has been used to relieve the valvular obstruction in selected cases using commissurotomy, combined with calcium debridement, either manually or with Cavitron ultrasonic aspiration.[34,35] Early experience indicated that these techniques reliably reduced the valvular gradient without inducing significant new aortic regurgitation.[34-36] Unfortunately, preliminary reports of follow-up of these patients have indicated unsatisfactory early postoperative results attributable to secondary fibrosis of the decalcified valve leaflets, producing significant aortic regurgitation and subsequent reoperation. Consequently, the number of patients currently undergoing aortic valve debridement has significantly dropped.

Aortic Regurgitation

Surgeons are showing increasing interest in applying the experience they have obtained with mitral valve repair to patients with severe aortic regurgitation and in attempting to repair, rather than replace, the aortic valve. The major interest has been focused on patients with isolated prolapse of one of the aortic valve leaflets, where the surgeon performs a wedge resection of the middle of the prolapsed leaflet, combined with an aortic annuloplasty. Successful operations have been performed in patients with tricuspid and bicuspid aortic valves.[37] Intraoperative TEE has been crucial in determining this mechanism of aortic regurgitation as well as in assessing the adequacy of valve repair (Fig. 16-16).

Aortic Homograft

There has been an increasing resurgence in the use of aortic homografts with the availability of cryopreserved aortic homograft valves. As with aortic valve

repair, this requires greater surgical expertise to perform aortic homograft replacement. Intraoperative TEE is an excellent tool that permits an approximation of the size of the aortic homograft needed, by measuring the aortic annular diameter. Immediately postinsertion, TEE provides the surgeon with an immediate assessment of the adequacy of insertion and can detect such complications as aortic regurgitation (central or perivalvular), hematoma formation, or left ventricular outflow tract obstruction.

Hypertrophic Obstructive Cardiomyopathy

In patients with hypertrophic obstructive cardiomyopathy who have substantial outflow tract gradients and refractory symptoms, relief of the outflow obstruction using transaortic septal myectomy may be warranted. Intraoperative echocardiography (TEE or epicardial echocardiography) is useful in these patients both before and after cardiopulmonary bypass (Figs. 16-17 and 16-18). The prebypass study permits a clear delineation of anatomy[38] and hemodynamics at baseline. These can be compared to postmyectomy studies at rest and with provacation with isoproterenol infusion. The distribution of left ventricular hy-

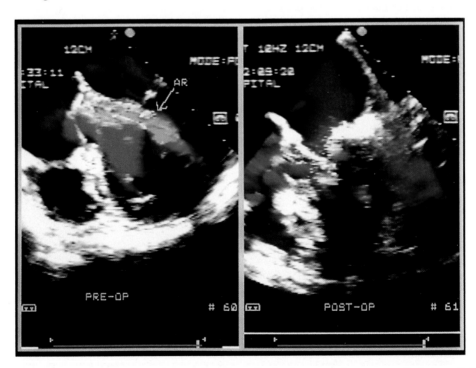

Fig. 16-16. Aortic regurgitation in a patient undergoing mitral valve repair for severe mitral regurgitation. The preoperative *(Left)* color Doppler study shows moderate aortic regurgitation (AR). After resuspension of a prolapsing noncoronary aortic valve cusp, the postoperative *(Right)* color Doppler study shows minimal aortic regurgitation.

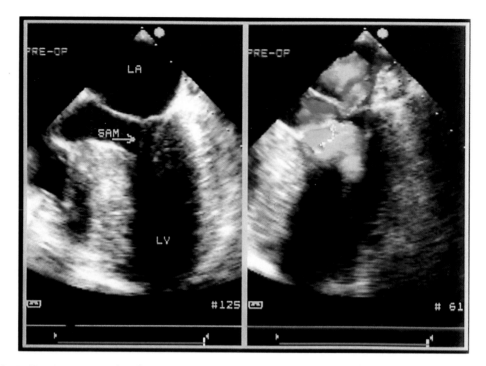

Fig. 16-17. Preoperative study of patient with hypertrophic obstructive cardiomyopathy. *(Left)* Transverse midesophageal plane showing hypertrophy of the ventricular septum and systolic anterior motion (SAM) of the mitral valve. *(Right)* Color Doppler showing mitral regurgitation and turbulent flow in the left ventricular outflow tract. LA, left atrium; LV, left ventricle.

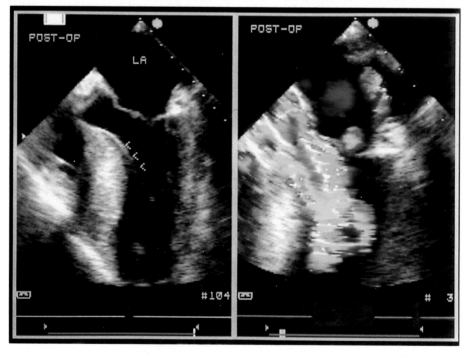

Fig. 16-18. Postoperative study of same patient shown in Figure 16-17. *(Left)* End-systolic freeze frame showing the region of septal myectomy (arrowheads). There is no systolic anterior motion of the mitral valve. *(Right)* Color Doppler showing mild residual mitral regurgitation. LA, left atrium.

pertrophy, the presence of hyperdynamic systolic function, systolic anterior motion of the mitral valve, and aortic valve midsystolic closure can be delineated. Color Doppler depicts the location of the high-velocity outflow tract jet emanating from the point of systolic apposition of the mitral valve against the ventricular septum.[39] It is helpful to the surgeon to determine the distance between this point of obstruction and the aortic annulus, to ensure that the myectomy is long enough. Color Doppler postseptal myectomy is helpful in assessing the severity of residual mitral regurgitation, in ensuring no significant aortic regurgitation, and in excluding the development of a ventricular septal defect from a too extensive myectomy. The mechanism of mitral regurgitation in these patients is typically related to the severity of systolic anterior motion of the mitral valve, hence the severity of left ventricular outflow tract obstruction. Continuous-wave Doppler is used to calculate the outflow tract gradient using the modified Bernoulli equation. If substantial resting or inducible obstruction persists, cardiopulmonary bypass can be reinstituted for further myectomy or mitral valve replacement.

Discrete Membranous Subaortic Stenosis

Left ventricular outflow tract obstruction may be caused by a discrete subaortic membrane. In some cases, the membrane is combined with a muscular tunnel as the cause of obstruction. Intraoperative TEE may be used to visualize the site of membranous left ventricular outflow tract obstruction. The extent of the membrane both before and after resection can be visualized. Continuous-wave Doppler velocity recordings can document the improvement in the outflow tract gradient. The presence and severity of aortic regurgitation can also be assessed by intraoperative TEE with color Doppler.

RETAINED INTRACARDIAC AIR

Another important intraoperative application of TEE is in the detection of air in the heart. Air bubbles are easily visualized by transesophageal scanning as numerous, small, highly reflective echo densities that float in the cardiac chambers (Fig. 16-19). In our experience, it is extremely common to find mobile intracardiac bubbles during open heart surgery; their

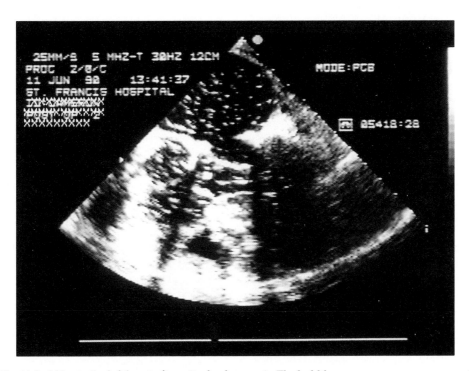

Fig. 16-19. Air bubbles in the left heart after mitral valve repair. The bubbles are seen as numerous, small, highly refrectile echo densities that float in the cardiac chambers and aorta.

frequent occurrence suggests that it is common for some air to gain access to the central circulation during open heart surgery. TEE readily demonstrates the presence of intracardiac air; however, quantitative assessment of air volume is impossible by this approach, and most patients with intracardiac air demonstrated by this method have no neurologic events. We recently encountered a patient who had difficulty coming off cardiopulmonary bypass. TEE demonstrated evidence of severe left ventricular systolic dysfunction, but the preoperative study had shown normal cardiac function. TEE demonstrated a large volume of air bubbles in the left cardiac chambers and was of help to the surgeon in de-airing the cardiac chambers. The patient was subsequently weaned off bypass.

Air embolism is a major risk in patients undergoing neurosurgical procedures and implantation of hip prostheses.[40] In one study, TEE demonstrated the presence of considerable air bubbles in the right atrium and right ventricle and of mild pulmonary emboli during the implantation of a femoral shaft prosthesis.[40] Paradoxical embolization is thought to occur through a patent foramen ovale.[41] Air embolism is also associated with other surgical procedures, including laparoscopy and cervical laminectomy.[20] TEE is the most sensitive monitor for intracardiac air and is the only effective monitoring device for paradoxic air embolism.

POTENTIAL ERRORS OF INTRAOPERATIVE ECHOCARDIOGRAPHY

The performance of intraoperative echocardiography requires an experienced echocardiographer who is familiar with echo and Doppler techniques, as well as with surgical repair procedures. Intraoperative echocardiography requires that images be interpreted on line so that surgical decisions can be made immediately. The intraoperative study requires precision, to ensure accuracy and reliability. Insufficient time, inadequate imaging planes, or suboptimal instrument machine settings will give less reliable information (Table 16-4). Electrocautery causes artifacts that interfere with image quality. The anesthesiologist, surgeon, and echocardiographer should

Table 16-4. Potential Errors of Intraoperative Echocardiography

Inexperienced echocardiographer
Suboptimal study
Limited imaging planes
Imaging time too short
Environmental factors
Room lights on
Electrocautery
Other forms of electrical interference
Hemodynamic instability
Hypotension
Hypothermia

be aware that the hemodynamic status of the patient should be optimized with pharmacologic manipulation of volume and afterload, to obtain an accurate assessment of any residual postrepair valvular regurgitation.

Most importantly, a team approach is needed for the optimal use of intraoperative TEE with the involvement of a cardiologist who has extensive echocardiographic expertise, an anesthesiologist, and a surgeon.

REFERENCES

1. Dahm M, Iversen S, Schmid FX, et al. Intraoperative evaluation of reconstruction of the atrioventricular valves by transesophageal echocardiography. J Thorac Cardiovasc Surg 1987; 35(special issue 2):140–142.
2. Drexler M, Erbel R, Dahm M, et al. Assessment of successful valve reconstruction by intraoperative transesophageal echocardiography (TEE). Int J Cardiac Imag 1986; 2:21–30.
3. Perier P, Deloche A, Chauvaud S, et al. Comparative evaluation of mitral valve repair and replacement with Starr, Bjork, and porcine valve prostheses. Circulation 1984; 70(suppl I):187–192.
4. Bonchek LI. Correction of mitral valve disease without mitral valve replacement. Am Heart J 1982; 104:865–868.
5. Goldman ME, Mora F, Fuster V, et al. Is mitral valvuloplasty superior to mitral valve replacement for preservation of left ventricular function? An intraoperative two-dimensional echocardiographic study. J Am Coll Cardiol 1986; 7(suppl A):161A (abst).
6. David TE, Uden DE, Strauss HD. The importance of the mitral apparatus in left ventricular function after correction of mitral regurgitation. Circulation 1983; 68(suppl II):76–82.
7. King R, Schaff H, Danielson G, et al. Surgery for tricuspid regurgitation late after mitral valve replacement. Circulation 1984; 70(suppl I):193–197.
8. Antunes MJ, Colsen PR, Kinsley RH. Mitral valvuloplasty: a learning curve. Circulation 1983; 68(suppl II):70–75.

9. Carpentier A, Chauvaud S, Fabiani JN, et al. Reconstructive surgery of mitral valve incompetence: ten year appraisal. J Thorac Cardiovasc Surg 1980; 79:338–348.
10. Mindich BP, Goldman ME. Intraoperative evaluation of valvular regurgitation: comparison of conventional and echocardiographic methods. In Maurer G, Mohl W (eds): Echocardiography and Doppler in Cardiac Surgery. New York: Igaku-Shoin, 1989, pp 227–242.
11. Maurer G, Czer L, Chaux A, et al. Intraoperative Doppler color flow mapping for assessment of valve repair for mitral regurgitation. Am J Cardiol 1987; 60:333–337.
12. Czer L, Maurer G, Bolger AF, et al. Intraoperative evaluation of mitral regurgitation by Doppler color flow mapping. Circulation 1987; 76(suppl III):108–116.
13. Czer L, Maurer G, Bolger A, et al. Tricuspid valve repair: operative and follow-up evaluation by Doppler color flow mapping. J Thorac Cardiovasc Surg 1989; 98:101–111.
14. Pagliero KM, Yates AK. Perioperative assessment of mitral valve function. J Thorac Cardiovasc Surg 1972; 63:458–460.
15. King H, Csicsko J, Leshnower A. Intraoperative assessment of the mitral valve following reconstructive procedures. Ann Thorac Surg 1980; 29:81–83.
16. Fuchs RM, Heuser RR, Yin FC, Brinker JA. Limitations of pulmonary wedge V-waves in diagnosing mitral regurgitation. Am J Cardiol 1982; 49:849–854.
17. Maurer G, Siegel RJ, Czer LSC. The use of color flow mapping for intraoperative assessment of valve repair. Circulation 1991; 84(suppl I):250–258.
18. Czer LSC, Maurer G, Bolger A, et al. Ischemic mitral regurgitation: comparative evaluation of revascularization versus repair by Doppler color flow mapping. Circulation 1987; 76(suppl IV):389.
19. Galler M, Kronzon I, Slater J, et al. Long-term follow-up after mitral valve reconstruction: incidence of postoperative left ventricular outflow obstruction. Circulation 1986; 74(suppl I):99.
20. Seward JB, Khandheria BK, Oh JK, et al. Transesophageal echocardiography: technique, anatomic correlations, implementation, and clinical applications. Mayo Clin Proc 1988; 63:649–680.
21. Kreindel MS. Systolic anterior motion of the mitral valve after Carpentier ring valvuloplasty for mitral valve prolapse. Am J Cardiol 1986; 57:408–414.
22. Marwick T. Echo evaluation of immediate and late failed mitral valve repair. J Am Coll Cardiol 1989; 13:114A (abst).
23. Mihaileanu S, Marino JP, Chauvaud S, et al. Left ventricular outflow obstruction after mitral valve repair (Carpentier's technique): proposed mechanisms of disease. Circulation 1988; 78(suppl I):78.
24. Schiavone WA, Cosgrove DM, Lever HM, et al. Long-term follow-up of patients with left ventricular outflow tract obstruction after Carpentier ring mitral valvuloplasty. Circulation 1988; 78(suppl I):60.
25. Currie PJ, Calafiore PA, Stewart WJ, et al. Transesophageal echo in mitral prosthetic dysfunction: echo-surgical correlation in 60 patients. J Am Coll Cardiol 1989; 13:69A (abstr).
26. Currie PJ. Transesophageal echocardiography: intraoperative applications. Echocardiography 1989; 6:403–414.
27. McAfee MK, Schaff HV. Valve repair for mitral insufficiency. Cardiology 1990; 7:35–43.
28. Marwick T, Currie PJ, Stewart WJ, et al. Echocardiographic evaluation of immediate and late failed mitral valve repair. J Am Coll Cardiol 1989; 13:114A (abst).
29. Koutlas TC, DeBruijn NP, Sheikh KH, et al. Chordal rupture as a late complication after mitral valve reconstruction. J Thorac Cardiovasc Surg 1991; 102:466–468.
30. Stewart WJ, Currie PJ, Lytle BW, et al. The role of intraoperative echocardiography in cardiac valvular surgery. J Am Coll Cardiol 1988; 11:217A (abst).
31. Wilkes HS, Berger M, Gallerstein PE, et al. Left ventricular outflow tract obstruction after aortic valve replacement: detection with continuous wave Doppler ultrasound recording. J Am Coll Cardiol 1983; 1:550–554.
32. Cutrone F, Coyle JP, Novoa R, et al. Severe dynamic left ventricular outflow tract obstruction following aortic valve replacement diagnosed by intraoperative echocardiography. Anesthesiology 1990; 72:563–569.
33. Stewart WJ, Currie PJ, Agler DA, et al. Periprosthetic mitral and aortic regurgitation: utility of pre- and intraoperative Doppler flow mapping. J Am Coll Cardiol 1988; 11:20A (abst).
34. Cosgrove DM, Gill CC, Lytle BW, et al. Aortic valvuloplasty in adults. Circulation 1987; 76(suppl IV):447 (abst).
35. Mindich BP, Guarino T, Kronz H, et al. Aortic valve salvage utilizing high frequency vibratory debridement. J Am Coll Cardiol 1988; 11:3A (abst).
36. Stewart WJ, Currie PJ, Salcedo EE, et al. Intraoperative echo in aortic valve repair. Circulation 1988; 78(suppl II):435 (abst).
37. Currie PJ, Stewart WJ. Intraoperative echocardiography for surgical repair of the aortic valve and left ventricular outflow tract. Echocardiography 1990; 7:273–288.
38. Syracuse DC, Caudiani VA, Kastl DC, et al. Intracardiac echocardiography during left ventricular myotomy and myectomy for hypertrophic subaortic stenosis. Circulation 1978; 58:23–30.
39. Stewart WJ, Schiavone WA, Salcedo EE, et al. Intraoperative Doppler echocardiography in hypertrophic cardiomyopathy: correlations with the obstructive gradient. J Am Coll Cardiol 1987; 10:327–335.
40. Ulrich C, Burri C, Wörsdörfer O, Heinrich H. Intraoperative transesophageal two-dimensional echocardiography in total hip replacement. Arch Orthop Trauma Surg 1986; 105:274–278.
41. Cucchiara RF, Seward JB, Nishimura RA, et al. Identification of patent foramen ovale during sitting position craniotomy by transesophageal echocardiography with positive air way pressure. Anesthesiology 1985; 63:107–109.

17 Intraoperative Monitoring of Ischemia and Systolic Cardiac Function

TERENCE RAFFERTY

The past decade has been marked by a trend from invasive to noninvasive intraoperative monitoring. As far as respiratory monitoring is concerned, initial experience with transcutaneous gas analysis laid the foundation for the widespread clinical use of pulse oximetry and end-tidal gas analysis. It has long been recognized that echocardiography might became an equally useful adjunct to cardiovascular monitoring. The disadvantages of transthoracic echocardiographic (TTE) imaging, including failure to depict cardiac structures adequately in many patients with obesity and emphysema, and constraints imposed by dressings and chest tubes, have limited the widespread application of the technique. Epicardial imaging, by necessity, requires an open chest and interferes with the surgical procedure. The transesophageal "window" does not suffer from these disadvantages. The site of data acquisition ("head of the table") makes TEE particularly applicable to an intraoperative setting (Fig. 17-1).

LEFT VENTRICULAR REGIONAL WALL-MOTION ABNORMALITIES

Detection of ischemia by two-dimensional echocardiography is based on the principle that acute myocardial ischemia results in deterioration of systolic function.[1] This is evidenced by the onset of wall-motion abnormalities and a decrease in systolic wall thickening.[2-9] Wall-motion abnormalities are considered present if the myocardium demonstrates minimal thickening or motion (hypokinesis), no thickening or motion (akinesis), or systolic thinning and paradoxic motion (dyskinesis). For the purposes of continuous monitoring, the most commonly employed view of the myocardium for TEE detection of ischemia is a transgastric transverse plane short-axis view of the left ventricle at the level of the papillary muscles[10-14] (Fig. 17-2). This view is selected because it contains portions of ventricular wall supplied by all three coronary arteries: the septum and anterior wall by the left anterior descending artery, the lateral wall by the circumflex marginal arteries, and the posterior wall by terminal branches of the right coronary artery. The corresponding longitudinal plane view, available with biplane endoscopy, permits visualization of the posteroinferior and anterolateral wall of the ventricle.[15,16]

The advent of coronary angioplasty has afforded clinical investigators the opportunity to study the time sequence of acute ischemia. The earliest association with coronary flow deprivation is the onset of two-dimensional echocardiographic regional wall-

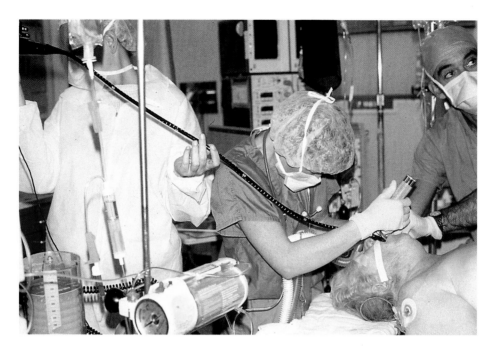

Fig. 17-1. Intraoperative insertion of a TEE endoscope.

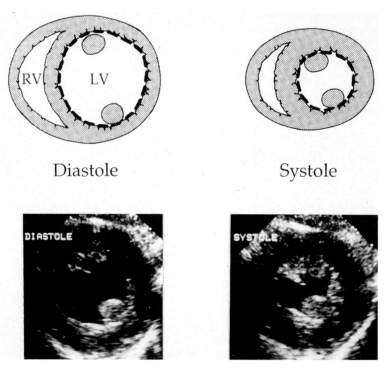

Fig. 17-2. Transgastric transverse plane left ventricular short axis papillary muscle level image. LV, left ventricle; RV, right ventricle. (From Rafferty,[151] with permission.)

Table 17-1. Relationship Between Angioplasty-Associated Coronary Flow Deprivation and the Onset of Regional Wall-Motion Abnormalties and ECG Changes

	Onset (s)	
	Wohlgelernter et al.[4]	Hauser et al.[5]
RWMA	10	19
ECG	22	30

Abbreviations: ECG: electrocardiogram; RWMA, regional wall-motion abnormalities.
(Modified from Rafferty,[151] with permission.)

motion abnormalities.[4,5] Electrocardiographic (ECG) changes follow after a variable latency period (Table 17-1). Angina is a relatively late presentation and, indeed, does not occur at all in approximately one-third of cases. If a comparison between 2-D echocardiography and ECG monitoring merely demonstrated differing latencies in the order of seconds, the issue might be considered trivial. However, in a separate publication that also pertained to findings established during angioplasty, Wohlgelernter et al.[6] also demonstrated a relative ischemia detection sensitivity of 2-D TTE, as compared with 3-lead and 12-lead ECG monitoring. These findings also pertain to transesophageal monitoring. Smith et al.[2] studied the relative sensitivities of standard ECG monitoring (leads I, II, III, aVR, aVL, aVF, and V5) and TEE regional wall-motion abnormalities as indicators of ischemia in vascular surgery and coronary artery bypass graft (CABG) patients. The investigators demonstrated an incidence of 24 new regional wall-motion abnormalities in 50 patients, while the corresponding incidence of new ST-segment changes was only six. In a similar study, Leung et al.[7] evaluated the relative sensitivities of Holter monitoring (modified V5 leads) and TEE for the detection of ischemia in CABG patients. These investigators noted that 82 percent of the regional wall-motion abnormalities in their patients were unassociated with corresponding Holter monitoring abnormalities. Furthermore, the advent of a regional wall-motion abnormality was predictive of outcome in this series (Fig. 17-3). None of 32 patients without regional wall-motion abnormalities suffered an adverse outcome. By contrast, 6 of 18 patients with postcardiopulmonary bypass

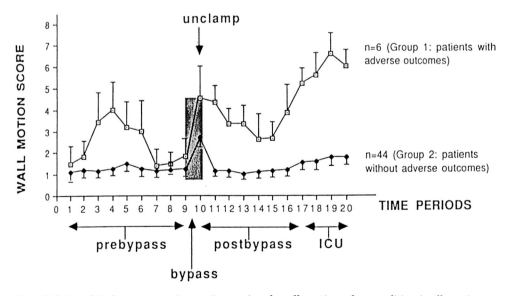

Fig. 17-3. Relationship between perioperative regional wall-motion abnormalities (wall-motion score) and outcome in coronary artery bypass graft patients. Increased score indicates increased regional wall-motion abnormalities. ICU, intensive care unit. (From Leung et al.,[7] with permission.)

graft regional wall-motion abnormalities had adverse outcomes (two deaths, three myocardial infarcts, and open congestive cardiac failure). Harris et al.[8] also monitored ST-segment changes (leads V5 and II) during CABG surgery. ST-segment changes occurred in 5 of 34 patients, while new regional wall-motion abnormalities occurred in 10 patients. Three of four postoperative myocardial infarctions correlated with antecedent regional wall-motion abnormalities, whereas only one was associated with intraoperative ECG changes.

In view of these data, one might reasonably question the propriety of using the electrocardiogram as a "gold standard" for ischemia. However, the use of regional wall-motion abnormalities as an alternate standard does have its pitfalls. There is a capacity for both false-negative and false-positive diagnoses. Leung et al.[7] and Harris et al.[8] documented three and six episodes, respectively, of ECG-defined ischemia in the absence of new regional wall-motion abnormalities. Similar findings were reported by London et al.[9] Such false-negative findings may have been due to ischemia in nonimaged areas, such as the left ventricular base or apex. Alternatively, observer variability may have played a role, a degree of variability being intrinsic to the technique. With regard to false-positive findings, it must be emphasized that technically inadequate images may predispose to an erroneous diagnosis. Inadequate endocardial definition or an oblique cross section precludes valid interpretation. Biologic variables must also be considered. Dyskinesia and akinesia are rare findings in normal subjects and may be considered reliable indicators of pathology. By contrast, hypokinesia is not specific for ischemia. Panadian et al.[17] showed that there is a wide range of normal contractile patterns, with significant segment to segment variability as a normal variant. A caveat is also applicable to analysis of septal motion in cases with cardiac systolic rotation and translational motion, these being particularly pronounced after sternotomy and pericardiectomy. In this situation, analysis with a center-of-mass reference may disclose apparent paradoxical motion.[18] Finally, true discoordinated contraction of the septum occurs in bundle-branch block and in association with ventricular pacing.

ASSESSMENT OF LEFT VENTRICULAR EJECTION FRACTION AND END-DIASTOLIC VOLUME

The accuracy of echocardiographic estimation of overall left ventricular ejection fraction and end-diastolic volume increases pari passu with the number of imaging planes taken into consideration.[19] However, the transesophageal "window" is limited in the number of imaging planes available. In addition, the left ventricular apex is commonly ill-defined by TEE, particularly in transverse plane longitudinal axis images. When the apex is visualized, it can be difficult to establish that the image is unassociated with an oblique angle of interrogation. A foreshortened image would furnish a significant underestimation of left ventricular dimensions. By contrast, transverse plane short-axis papillary muscle level images are reliably reproducible. The absence of interrogation angle obliquity can be inferred from the quality of papillary muscle outlines. Several investigators have evaluated the relationship between cross-sectional measurements of the left ventricle and "gold standard" estimates of ejection fraction and volume status. Clements et al.[20] studied 12 patients during abdominal aortic aneurysm surgery, with the transducer maintained at midpapillary muscle level throughout the procedures. At multiple times during surgery, echocardiograms and first-pass radionuclide angiograms were recorded simultaneously. The correlation between planimetered area fractional shortening and corresponding radionuclide ejection fraction measurements was close ($r = 0.96$) (Fig. 17-4). There was also a significant relationship between diastolic planimetered area and radionuclide end-diastolic volume estimates ($r = 0.85$) (Fig. 17-5). Interestingly, the relationship between the extent of systolic cavity obliteration and corresponding end-systolic radionuclear estimates was even closer ($r = 0.92$) (Fig. 17-6), perhaps on the basis of clearer endocardial definition during systole. Urbanowitz et al.[21] studied 10 cardiac surgery patients using a blood pool scintigraphy/thermodilution cardiac output standard. Again, there was a close correlation between planimetered area fractional shortening and the reference method ejection fraction ($r = 0.82$)

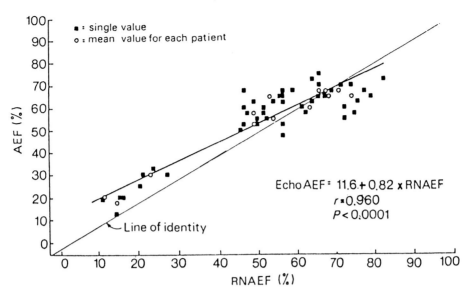

Fig. 17-4. Correlation between transgastric transverse plane left ventricular short-axis ejection fraction measurements and ejection fraction determined by first-pass radionuclide angiography. Data are expressed as logarithms. AEF, axis ejection fraction; RNAEF, radionuclide axis ejection fraction. (From Clements et al.,[20] with permission.)

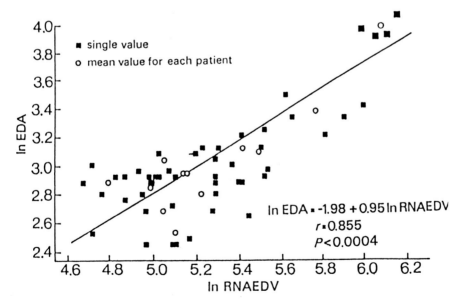

Fig. 17-5. Correlation between transgastric transverse plane left ventricular short-axis end-diastolic planimetered area and first-pass radionuclide angiographic measurements of end-diastolic volume (RNAEDV). Data are expressed as logarithms. EDA, end-diastolic area. (From Clements et al.,[20] with permission.)

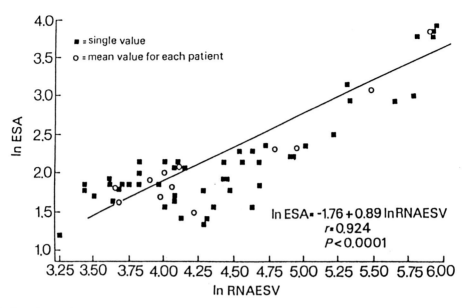

Fig. 17-6. Correlation between transgastric transverse plane left ventricular short-axis end-systolic planimetered area (ESA) and first-pass radionuclide angiographic measurements of end-systolic volume (RNAESV). Data are expressed as logarithms. (From Clements et al.,[20] with permission.)

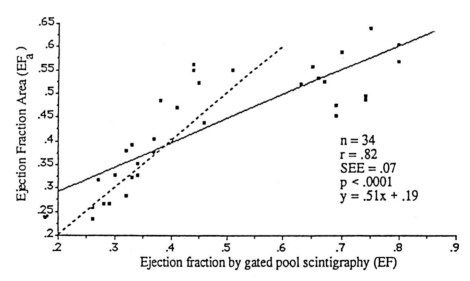

Fig. 17-7. Correlation between transgastric transverse plane left ventricular short-axis ejection fraction measurements and ejection fraction determined by blood pool scintigraphy/thermodilution cardiac output techniques. (From Urbanowitz et al.,[21] with permission.)

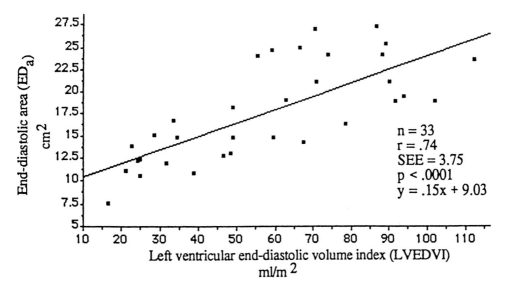

Fig. 17-8. Correlation between transgastric transverse plane left ventricular short-axis end-diastolic planimetered area and blood pool scintigraphy/thermodilution cardiac output technique measurements of end-diastolic volume. (From Urbanowitz et al.,[21] with permission.)

(Fig. 17-7). Comparison of end-diastolic area measurements and calculated end-diastolic volume estimates also demonstrated a significant relationship ($r = 0.74$) (Fig. 17-8). However, discordant changes were observed in three patients (a frequency of 17 percent), and the Urbanowitz et al. recommended that such transesophageal data be used only to determine rather large differences in volume status.

AUTOMATED ENDOCARDIAL OUTLINE DETECTION

Recent advances in technology have brought automated detection of blood-tissue interfaces into the clinical realm. In this context, the blood-tissue interface is the outline of the endocardium. This so-called "acoustic quantification technique" can circumvent the necessity for time-consuming manual planimetry of diastolic and systolic endocardial cross-sectional outlines when it comes to measurement of ventricular cavity areas. This raises the possibility of on-line measurement and display of echocardiographic estimates of volume status and ejection fraction. Prelimi-

nary data have shown a close correlation between measurements derived from these automated systems and estimates derived by standard laboratory methods, at least with high-resolution images.[22-29] The clinical utility of this technique for continuous monitoring remains to be determined.

RIGHT VENTRICULAR SYSTOLIC PERFORMANCE INDICES

Tricuspid Annular Plane Systolic Excursion

Transesophageal transverse plane imaging permits simultaneous visualization of the lateral border of the tricuspid annulus and the right ventricular free wall-septal junction. This view is reproducibly provided by the longitudinal axis plane transecting the ventricle from base to apex below the level of the aortic valve and above the level of the coronary sinus[30] (Fig. 17-9). The coronary sinus view is presented for comparison (Fig. 17-10). The right ventricular major axis in this view is considered to be represented by a line drawn from the apex to bisect the midannular plane

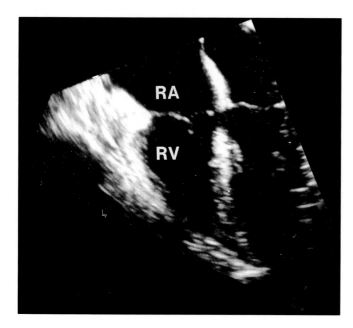

Fig. 17-9. Transesophageal transverse plane long-axis image of the right ventricle determined at the level of the anterior mitral leaflet. RA, right atrium; RV, right ventricle.

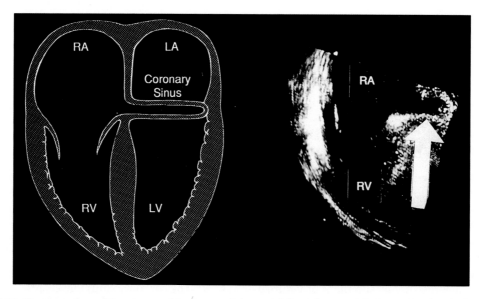

Fig. 17-10. Transesophageal transverse plane long-axis image of the right ventricle determined at the level of the coronary sinus (arrow). Noted that the apex of the ventricle cannot be visualized. LA, left atrium; LV, left ventricle; RA, right atrium; RV, right ventricle.

of the tricuspid valve. The maximal major axis is more lateral in orientation and connects the apex of the ventricle to the lateral border of the annulus. The amplitude of motion from end-diastole to end-systole represents the excursion of this latter annular border.[31,32] This segmental contractility measurement was first proposed by Kaul et al.[31] under the nomenclature of tricuspid annular plane systolic excursion (TAPSE). These investigators demonstrated a close correlation ($r = 0.92$) between transthoracic determinations of TAPSE and right ventricular ejection fraction measurements obtained by radionuclide angiography. In this series, annular motion was expressed as an absolute dimension rather than as a systolic/diastolic ratio. A subsequent interpretation of the measurement method inferred apical delineation as part of the technique[33] (Fig. 17-11). Finally, the expression of the longitudinal maximal major axis shortening fraction measurements as a ratio allows for facile data intercomparison.[30,34,35]

Maximal Minor Axis Shortening Fraction

The corresponding transverse plane longitudinal minor axis of the right ventricle is the distance between the free wall and septum in a plane perpendicular to the major axis.[33] The maximal minor axis lies close to the tricuspid valve, being displaced inferiorly in cases of volume overload.[36] The maximal minor axis shortening fraction has been proposed as a logical right ventricular contractility index[33] (Fig. 17-12). Transesophageal determinations of this measurement are reproducible and comparable in accuracy to right ventricular planimetered area excursion fraction measurements.[37] Maximal minor axis shortening fraction measurements may be directly affected by dysfunction of the interventricular septum. Paradoxical septal motion, being a left ventricular systolic correction of diastolic right ventricular displacement of the septum into the left ventricular cavity, would be anticipated to result in an exaggeration of the systolic excursion of the maximal minor axis. This would be expected to generate a shortening fraction value directly reflecting right and left ventricular performance, as well as the transseptal pressure gradient. However, there are no available data pertaining to this issue.

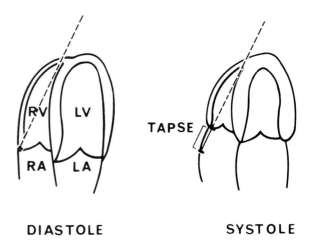

Fig. 17-11. Schematic representation of tricuspid annular plane systolic excursion. LA, left atrium; LV, left ventricle; RA, right atrium; RV, right ventricle; TAPSE, tricuspid annular plane systolic excursion. (From Feigenbaum,[33] with permission.)

Right Ventricular Planimetered Area Excursion Fraction

Transthoracic longitudinal axis right ventricular planimetered area measurements have been shown to be reliably reproducible.[38] Such excursion fraction measurements have been gainfully employed to study the hemodynamic effects of positive end-expiratory pressure (PEEP).[39] Corresponding trans-

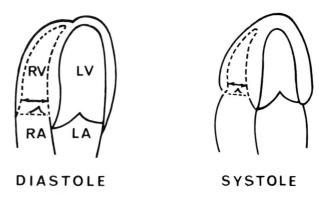

Fig. 17-12. Schematic representation of maximal minor axis shortening fraction. LA, left atrium; LV, left ventricle; RA, right atrium; RV, right ventricle. (From Feigenbaum,[33] with permission.)

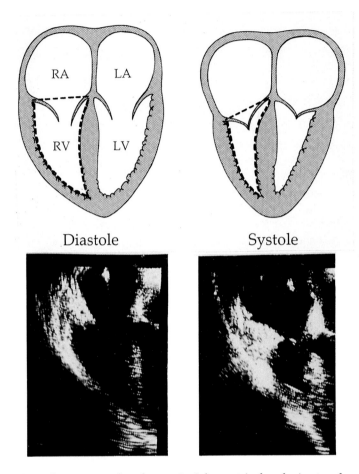

Fig. 17-13. Transesophageal transverse plane long-axis right ventricular planimetered area excursion fraction. LA, left atrium; LV, left ventricle; RA, right atrium; RV, right ventricle.

esophageal data are limited to evaluation of transverse plane image reproducibility at differing levels of interrogation. Durkin and co-workers[30,37] contrasted longitudinal axis planimetered area excursion fraction measurements (Fig. 17-13) with tricuspid annular plane systolic excursion ratio and maximal minor axis shortening fraction in the intact and open chest. These investigators reported that the right ventricular coronary sinus level view was inconsistent with coincident imaging of the tricuspid annulus and right ventricular apex. Durkin's group recommended that the superiorly located anterior mitral leaflet be taken as the independent reference structure (Fig.

17-10). Bland-Altman bias analyses demonstrated that differences between measurements did not vary systematically over the measurement range (Figs. 17-14 and 17-15). Koorn et al.[40] contrasted planimetered area excursion fraction measurements with thermodilution measurements of right ventricular ejection fraction. These investigators reported a significant correlation ($r = 0.76$) between the variables. The bias distribution scatterplot was similar to the above figures. Because the echocardiographic absolute values overestimated "actual" right ventricular ejection, it was recommended that the technology be used as a trend monitor.

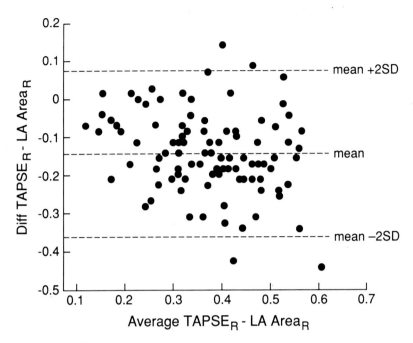

Fig. 17-14. The relationship (Bland-Altman analysis) between transesophageal transverse plane long-axis right ventricular planimetered area excursion fraction and corresponding tricuspid annular plane systolic excursion ratio measurements. LA area$_R$, longitudinal axis planimetered area excursion fraction; TAPSE$_R$, tricuspid annular plane systolic excursion ratio.

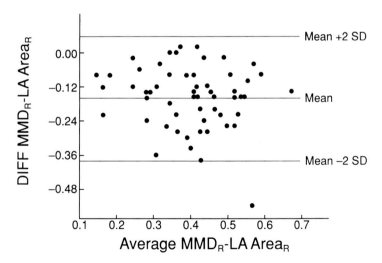

Fig. 17-15. The relationship (Bland-Altman analysis) between transesophageal transverse plane long-axis right ventricular planimetered area excursion fraction and corresponding maximal minor axis shortening fraction. LA area$_R$, longitudinal axis planimetered area excursion fraction; MMD$_R$, maximal minor axis shortening fraction. (From Durkin and Rafferty,[37] with permission.)

INTRAOPERATIVE APPLICATION

Two-dimensional TTE has been used to delineate changes in right ventricular regional wall-motion during exercise stress testing for more than a decade. In this context, Maurer and Nanda[41] reported their results in terms of a qualitative grading system, whereby cross sections were divided into three equal segments, and wall motion classified as normal or abnormal (hypokinetic, akinetic or dyskinetic). An illustrative four-chamber view cross section is presented in Figure 17-16. Analogous studies pertaining to analysis of intraoperative right ventricular function are not available.

Measurement of 2-D TTE systolic performance indices in multiple planes may find application in the delineation of intraoperative regional dysfunction by the following rationale. Two-dimensional echocardiographic shortening fraction and planimetered area excursion fraction measurements, by definition,

only measure function of individual right ventricular segments, irrespective of their correlation with independent estimates of global ejection fraction in given situations. A dynamic change in the interrelationships of the echocardiographic measurements could be interpreted as indicating regional inhomogeneity of performance, given a constant geometry and standardization of image acquisition technique, and consequent constant plane of interrogation.[35] However, few data exist on this issue.

MITRAL REGURGITATION

Transesophageal color Doppler evidence of mitral regurgitation is commonly observed in adult patients undergoing cardiac surgery. An unreported analysis of our patients demonstrated a 61 percent incidence of this finding in uncomplicated CABG patients. Overestimation of actual regurgitant volume by color Doppler mapping is well documented.[42-44] A finding of mild degrees of mitral regurgitation does not have significant adverse prognostic implications. However, recent preliminary data indicate that moderate and severe degrees of dysfunction do impact on short-term cardiac events and mortality rates.[45]

Color Doppler imaging of mitral regurgitation involves consideration of a variety of technical issues. Standardization of image acquisition techniques is important for valid intercomparison of data. It is well recognized that variations in instrument and instrument settings (e.g., pulse repetition frequency, gain settings, and interrogation depth) can markedly influence visually perceived regurgitant jet dimensions.[46-49] In addition, there is no uniformly accepted standard for quantification. Commonly employed methods can be divided into two categories: those involving measurement of regurgitant jet length and planimetered area, respectively, with or without concurrent pulsed-Doppler evaluation of pulmonary venous flow, each having its own inherent limitations. A compendium of published grading systems[50-57] is presented in Tables 17-2 to 17-4.

A listing of studies detailing the relationship between color Doppler and angiographic estimates of mitral regurgitation is presented in Tables 17-5 to 17-7. Comparison of these studies is complicated by differences in severity grading systems of regurgitation and

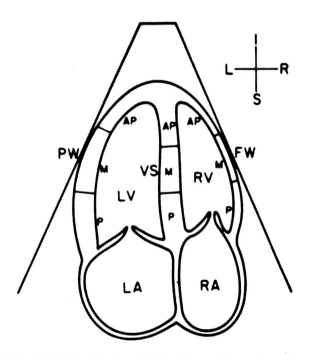

Fig. 17-16. Exercise stress testing demarcation system for qualitative analysis of right ventricular regional wall motion. A, anterior; FW, free wall; LA, left atrium; LV, left ventricle; M, mid; P, posterior; PW, posterior wall; RA, right atrium; RV, right ventricle; VS, ventricular septum. (From Maurer and Nanda,[41] with permission.)

Table 17-2. Grading of Mitral Regurgitation by Assessment of the Regurgitant Jet Depth of Atrial Penetration

Author	Grade 1	Grade 2	Grade 3	Grade 4
Omoto et al.[68]	<Middle of MV orifice and ring	<Level of MV ring	≤2 cm beyond MV ring	>2 cm beyond MV ring
Miyatake et al.[50]	<1.5 cm beyond MV orifice	<3 cm beyond MV orifice	<4.5 cm beyond MV orifice	≥4.5 cm beyond MV orifice
Maurer et al.[51]	Immediately below atrial aspect of MV	≤1.3 LA	≤2/3 LA	>2/3 LA
Czer et al.[52] Reichert et al.[53]				
Mohr-Kahaly et al.[54]	<2 cm (mild)	≤4 cm (moderate)	>4 cm (severe)	

Abbreviations: LA, Left atrium; MV, mitral valve.

Table 17-3. Grading of Mitral Regurgitation by Assessment of the Regurgitant Jet Area

Author	Mild	Moderate	Severe
Spain et al.[55]	<4 cm²	≤8 cm²	>8 cm²
Mohr-Kahaly et al.[54]	<3 cm²	≤6 cm²	>6 cm²
Nellessen et al.[56]	≤2 cm²	≤4 cm²	>4 cm²

Table 17-4. Grading of Mitral Regurgitation by Assessment of the Regurgitant Jet Area/ Left Atrial Area Ratio

Author	Mild	Moderate	Severe
Helmcke et al.[57] Spain et al.[55]	<0.20	≤0.40	>0.40
Mohr-Kahaly et al.[54]	<0.15	≤0.30	>0.30

statistical analysis techniques. In many of these studies, the raw data are available in the text. This made it possible to perform a spectrum of analyses, denoted in the appropriate tables by parentheses. Several series do contrast quantification methods. Spain et al.[55] reported that maximal jet area absolute values correlated more closely with angiographic grade than did values corrected for left atrial dimensions, i.e., maximal jet area/left atrial area ratio ($r = 0.76$ versus 0.71). Similar findings were observed by Mohr-Kahaly et al.[54] ($r = 0.81$ versus 0.77). By contrast, Helmeke et al.[57] reported their optimal correlation as being associated with left atrial dimension referenced measurements. Both of these latter groups did concur with respect to demonstrating a suboptimal correlation between regurgitant jet length mea-

Table 17-5. Mitral Regurgitant Jet Depth of Atrial Penetration as a Function of Angiographic Grade[a]

Author	Study Design	No. of Patients	Spearman Rank Coefficient	KAPPA
Omoto et al.[68] (TT)	Prospective	42	(0.91)	(0.83)
Miyatake et al.[50] (TT)	Prospective	109	0.87	(0.55)
Czer et al.[52] (epicardial)	Prospective	68	(0.90)	0.80
Maurer et al.[56] (TT)	Prospective	56	(0.88)	0.75
Maurer et al.[56] (epicardial)	Prospective	56	(0.89)	0.80
Helmcke et al.[57] (TT)	Combined retrospective/ prospective	82	--	--
Mohr-Kahaly et al.[54] (TT)	Prospective	42	0.81	(0.75)
Reichert et al.[53] (TEE pre-CPB)	Prospective	23	(0.84)	(0.90)
Reichert et al.[53] (TEE post-CPB)	Prospective	23	0.83	--

Abbreviations: CPB, cardiopulmonary bypass; TEE, transesophageal transverse plane; TT, transthoracic.
[a] Numbers in parentheses are calculated from raw data derived from the text; the dashed line represents data not extractable. Data expressed as sensitivity, specificity, and (positive) predictive value for each grade vis à vis corresponding angiographic grade (ranges of 93–94, 96–100, and 85–100 percent, respectively).

Table 17-6. Mitral Regurgitant Jet Area as a Function of Angiographic Grade[a]

Author	Study Design	No. of Patients	Spearman Rank Coefficient	KAPPA
Helmcke et al.[57] (TT)	Combined retrospective/prospective	47	0.76	--
Spain et al.[55] (TT)	Retrospective	42	--	--
Mohr-Kahaly et al.[54] (TT)	Prospective	42	0.81	(0.75)
Nelessen et al.[56] (TT)	Prospective	13	(0.60)	(0.24)
Nelessen et al.[56] (TEE)	Prospective	13	(1.00)	(0.84)

Abbreviations: CPB, cardiopulmonary bypass; TT, transthoracic; TEE, transesophageal transverse plane.
[a]Numbers in parentheses are calculated from raw data derived from the text; the dashed line represents data not extractable.

surements and angiographic grade. Finally, Mohr-Kahaly et al.[54] reported that the only clear separation between mild and severe regurgitation in their series was for the parameter derived from multiplying the absolute area of the jet by duration of regurgitation.

Sahn has reviewed factors that must be borne in mind when interpreting the depth of penetration of regurgitant jets into a receiving chamber.[58] Jet intrusion distance varies as a function of velocity times regurgitant orifice diameter. When the flow curves around or strikes a boundary, energy losses occur asymmetrically, tending to keep the jet adjacent to the boundary as it decelerates because of loss of energy to viscous friction. Finally, when a jet is struck by a fluid stream proceeding parallel to it or directed against it, as can occur with pulmonary venous inflow, deviation of jet direction occurs.[59] This is followed by breakup with a shortening of intrusion distance. The presence of restriction of the regurgitant orifice can have the opposite effect, and may result in a nozzle phenomenon, dissociating depth of jet penetration from severity of regurgitation.[60]

Regurgitant jet area measurements also have drawbacks. It is generally accepted that representative dimensions are those associated with a transducer orientation consistent with imaging of the maximal jet area. However, mitral regurgitant jets exhibit a wide spectrum of vectors, and it may not be possible to define the true maximal area by TEE, particularly when biplane interrogation capabilities are not available. Certainly, comparison of maximal jet area data obtained from transesophageal transverse and longitudinal planes demonstrates a nonuniform distribution of values.[61] In addition, the expression of mitral regurgitant jet area as a function of left atrial dimensions may not be applicable to transesophageal measurements. The bulk of the left atrial wall cannot be reliably imaged in most patients, even under conditions of cardiopulmonary bypass with associated extremes of decompression. Interpolation of nonvisualized boundaries, of necessity, involves a degree of inaccuracy.

Other factors must also be considered in evaluating regurgitant lesions. Wong et al.[62] demonstrated a bio-

Table 17-7. Mitral Regurgitant Jet Area/Left Atrial Area Ratio as a Function of Angiographic Grade[a]

Author	Study Design	No. of Patients	Spearman Rank Coefficient	KAPPA
Helmcke et al.[57] (TT)	Combined retrospective/prospective	82	--	--
Spain et al.[55] (TT)	Retrospective	47	0.71	--
Mohr-Kahaly et al.[54] (TT)	Prospective	42	0.77	(0.71)

Abbreviations: CPB, cardiopulmonary bypass; TEE, transesophageal transverse plane; TT, transthoracic.
[a]Numbers in parentheses are calculated from raw data derived from the text; the dashed line represents data not extractable.

logic source of variability, in that jet areas vary over a considerable portion of regurgitant flow time. Mitral jets reach maximal size at 12 percent to 75 percent into systole and at a mean of 35 percent of flow time. Furthermore, among five consecutive beats, regurgitant jet areas showed a consistent variability of 14 percent to 22 percent. Even when comparisons were made on identical frames, the subjectiveness of color edge detection is such that interobserver variability is as high as 15 percent.

AORTIC REGURGITATION

Preoperative screening of cardiac surgery patients does not routinely include aortographic assessment of aortic regurgitation in the absence of clinical manifestations of a disorder. The prevalence of aortic valve dysfunction in the general population is age related, and investigators have reported an 89 percent incidence of transthoracic Doppler-defined aortic regurgitation by the eighth decade.[63] Recent data suggest that the esophagus offers a satisfactory transducer orientation relative to the left ventricular outflow tract for aortic regurgitation measurements.[64–66] For these reasons, the routine use of intraoperative color Doppler monitoring in a predominantly elderly population, such as CABG patients, would be expected to be associated with a high incidence of previously unrecognized aortic regurgitation, albeit trivial in most instances.

Several investigators have defined a relationship between the severity of dysfunction and the depth of regurgitant jet penetration into the left ventricular cavity. In a color Doppler study, Miyatake et al.[67] noted that "the regurgitant flow reached the apical cavity in patients with severe aortic regurgitation." In a systematic analysis of this issue, Omoto et al.[68] demonstrated a significant relationship between color Doppler penetration grade and angiographic regurgitation grade. By contrast, Perry et al.[69] found no correlation between color Doppler jet length and angiographic grade and noted that several patients with a mild grade of aortic regurgitation had "a narrow regurgitant jet that extended deep into the left ventricle." Finally, in an in vitro model, Switzer et al.[70] reported that, while jet penetration depth accurately predicted peak flow velocity, it could not reliably predict orifice size.

An alternative quantification method is available. In the previously alluded-to prosthetic valve model, Switzer et al.[70] demonstrated that the color Doppler width of a regurgitant jet reliably predicts defect size. Perry et al.[69] confirmed the clinical applicability of such a measurement determined through a parasternal approach. These investigators expressed the proximal width of regurgitant jets as a function of the immediate receiving chamber dimensions (i.e., left ventricular outflow tract diameter). This technique is also applicable to transesophageal interrogation. Figure 17-17, a computer-aided 3-D representation of the aortic valve and left ventricular outflow tract, is

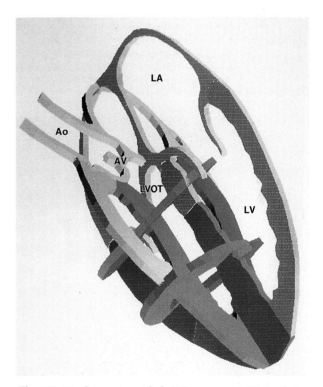

Fig. 17-17. Computer-aided 3-D representation of the heart orientated to illustrate the left ventricular outflow tract (LVOT). Ao, aorta; LA, left atrium; LV, left ventricle; LVOT, left ventricular outflow tract (Modified and reproduced courtesy of Lynch P, Jaffe C: Departments of Biomedical Communications and Diagnostic Radiology, Yale University School of Medicine.)

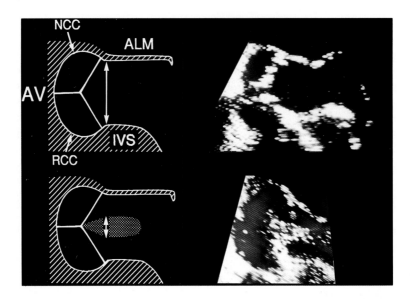

Fig. 17-18. Aortic regurgitation quantification technique. The proximal diameter of the regurgitant jet is expressed as a fraction of the corresponding left ventricular outflow tract diameter. Superimposition of color Doppler M-mode interrogation facilitates precision of measurements. ALM, anterior mitral leaflet; AV, aortic valve; IVS, interventricular septum; LVOT, left ventricular outflow tract; NCC, noncoronary cusp; RCC, right coronary cusp. (Modified from Rafferty et al.,[66] with permission.)

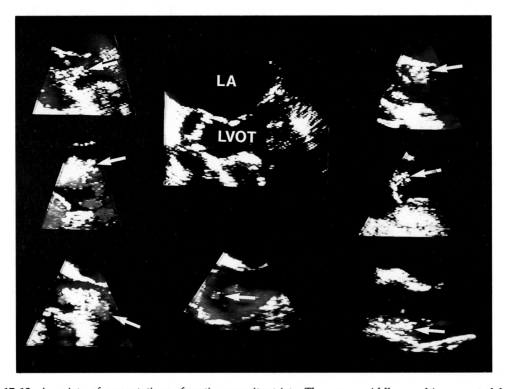

Fig. 17-19. A variety of presentations of aortic regurgitant jets. The upper middle panel is presented for the purpose of orientation. LA, left atrium; LVOT, left ventricular outflow tract. (From Rafferty et al.,[66] with permission.)

presented for the purposes of orientation. Figure 17-18 represents the above quantification technique. Superimposition of color Doppler M-mode interrogation facilitates precision of measurements. A variety of clinical presentations of aortic regurgitation are depicted in Figure 17-19.

TRICUSPID VALVE

The tricuspid valve can be reliably imaged in transesophageal transverse and longitudinal planes. Standard transverse plane longitudinal axis views are registered in a cross section transecting the ventricle from base to apex with the anterior mitral leaflet in the far field (see Fig. 17-9) and at the coronary sinus level (see Fig. 17-10). The standard longitudinal plane view of the valve is in a plane consistent with simultaneous visualization of the aortic root (Fig. 17-20).

COLOR DOPPLER TRICUSPID REGURGITATION

The prevalence of transthoracic pulsed Doppler-defined tricuspid regurgitation in normal subjects has been reported to be as high as 93 percent.[71] The upper

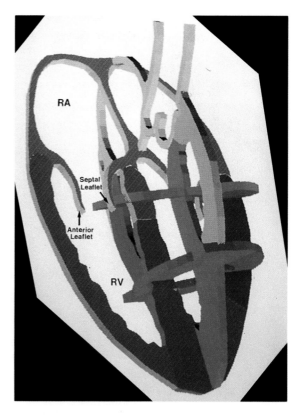

Fig. 17-21. Computer-aided 3-D representation of the heart orientated to illustrate the tricuspid valve. RA, right atrium; RV, right ventricle. (Modified and reproduced courtesy of Lynch P, Jaffe C: Departments of Biomedical Communications and Diagnostic Radiology, Yale University School of Medicine.)

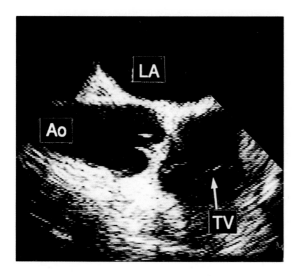

Fig. 17-20. Two-dimensional TEE longitudinal plane view of the tricuspid valve obtained with a biplane probe. Ao, aorta; LA, left atrium; TV, tricuspid valve.

limits of "normal" for transthoracic pulsed-Doppler tricuspid regurgitation have been variously defined as a regurgitant jet length of less than 1 cm and a regurgitant jet length of up to one-third of corresponding right atrial superoinferior dimensions, respectively.[72,73] Upper limits of "normal" for transthoracic color Doppler estimates have been reported as a regurgitant jet planimetered area of 1.52 cm².[73] Transesophageal color Doppler normalcy limits have been designated as a regurgitant jet area of 0.3 cm² and a jet area/right atrial area ratio of 4 percent, respectively, using saline-contrast evaluation of valve integrity as a comparative reference standard.[74,75] Figure 17-21, a computer-aided 3-D representation of the tricuspid valve, is presented for the

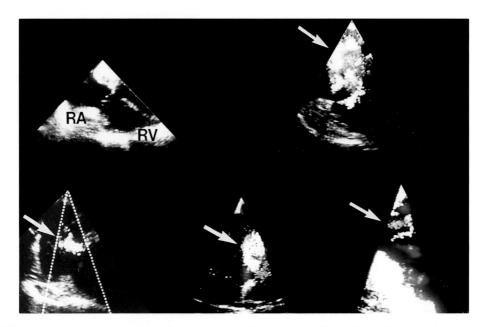

Fig. 17-22. A variety of presentations of transesophageal transverse plane views of tricuspid regurgitant jets. RA, right atrium; RV, right ventricle.

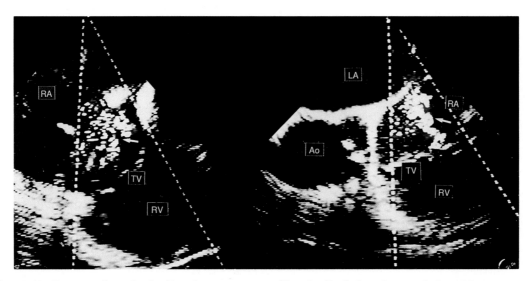

Fig. 17-23. Transesophageal color Doppler transverse and longitudinal plane image of tricuspid regurgitation. Arrow represents tricuspid regurgitation. Ao aorta; LA, left atrium; RA, right atrium; RV, right ventricle.

purposes of orientation. Figure 17-22 depicts a variety of clinical presentations of transverse plane tricuspid regurgitant jets. Figure 17-23 illustrates transverse and longitudinal plane views of tricuspid regurgitation.

Demographic data pertaining to the perioperative characteristics of tricuspid regurgitant jets are not available. The tricuspid valve leaflet apparatus, unlike that of the mitral valve, has insertion sites that relate to the intraventricular septum as well as the ventricular free wall. Thus, it might reasonably be speculated that tricuspid regurgitation could occur de novo or be exacerbated by ischemia-related dysfunction of widely separated regions of the myocardium. Transient increases in color Doppler jet area are not uncommon during the immediate postcardiopulmonary bypass period and may provide a method for intraoperative detection and quantification of ischemia.

A number of systems have been employed to estimate the severity of valve dysfunction. Miyatake et al.[71] classified the regurgitation according to the extent of right atrial penetration, with the atrium divided into four equal segments, graded 1+ to 4+, respectively. Takamoto et al.[76] have used a similar system, with the addition of an extracardiac measurement reflecting flow in the inferior vena cava. The degree of tricuspid regurgitation has also been quantified by cross-sectional area measurements, either as absolute planimetered area or in terms of the area expressed as a function of corresponding right atrial dimensions. These grading systems are represented schematically in Figures 17-24 and 17-25.

PULMONIC VALVE

The main pulmonary artery and its bifurcation can often be well visualized via the transesophageal transverse plane (Fig. 17-26). This finding does not apply to the pulmonic valve. In contrast, the longitudinal plane affords a more consistent view of this structure (Fig. 17-27). This latter "window" can be helpful intraoperatively as a means of delineating flow-directed pulmonary artery catheter position. A

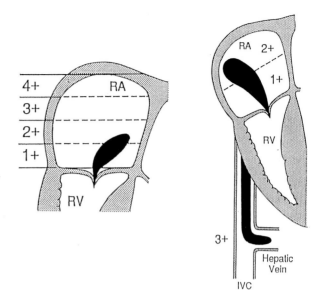

Fig. 17-24. Schematic representation of the quantification of tricuspid regurgitation in terms of regurgitant jet depth of retrograde penetration into the right atrium and inferior vena cava. *(Left)* Tricuspid regurgitant jet depth of right atrial retrograde penetration. *(Right)* Analogous severity of dysfunction grading system with the addition of an extracardiac index (inferior vena cava extension). IVC, inferior vena cava; RA, right atrium; RV, right ventricle.

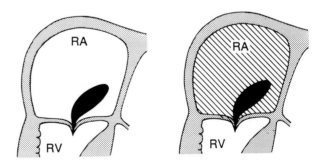

Fig. 17-25. Schematic representation of the quantification of tricuspid regurgitation in terms of regurgitant jet planimetered absolute cross-sectional area an area expressed as a function of right atrial area, respectively. *(Left)* Tricuspid regurgitant jet area. *(Right)* Tricuspid regurgitant jet area/right atrial area ratio. RA, right atrium; RV, right ventricle.

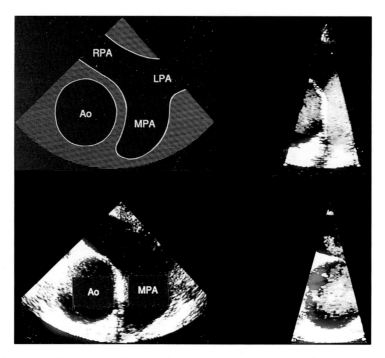

Fig. 17-26. Two-dimensional TEE and color Doppler transverse plane image of the pulmonary artery. *(Upper left)* Schematic representation of the main pulmonary artery (MPA) and right and left pulmonary arteries (RPA and LPA, respectively). *(Bottom left)* Two-dimensional echocardiographic image of the aorta (Ao), main pulmonary artery (MPA), right pulmonary artery, and origin of the left pulmonary artery. *(Upper right)* Color Doppler image of the MPA and aorta (Ao). *(Bottom right)* Color Doppler image of the aorta and right pulmonary artery.

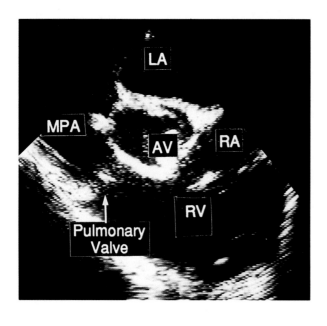

Fig. 17-27. Two-dimensional TEE longitudinal plane view of the pulmonic valve obtained with a biplane probe. AV, aortic valve; LA, left atrium; MPA, main pulmonary artery; RA, right atrium; RV, right ventricle.

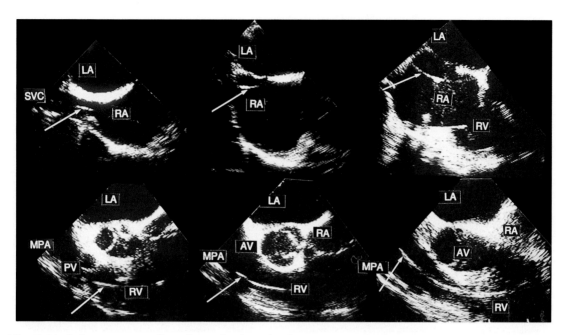

Fig. 17-28. Pulmonary artery flow-directed catheter localization using a biplane probe. *(Upper left)* Longitudinal plane view of catheter proximal to superior vena cava-right atrial junction. *(Upper middle)* Transverse plane view of catheter distal to the superior vena cava-right atrial junction. *(Upper right)* Transverse plane view of catheter at mid-right atrial level. *(Bottom left)* Longitudinal plane view of catheter just proximal to pulmonic valve. *(Bottom middle)* Longitudinal plane view of catheter in the proximal main pulmonary artery. *(Bottom right)* Longitudinal plane view of the catheter in the main pulmonary artery. AV, aortic valve; LA, left atrium; MPA, main pulmonary artery; PV, pulmonic valve; RA, right atrium; RV, right ventricle; SVC, superior vena cava.

guided sequence illustrating catheter passage from the superior vena cava to the main pulmonary artery is presented in Figure 17-28.

ASSESSMENT OF SURGICAL INTERVENTIONS

TEE has been widely used for intraoperative detailed evaluation of congenital cardiac disease.[77-82] Dan et al.[83] reported how the technique was employed to detect a partial detachment of the pericardial baffle in a modified Fontan procedure patient who manifested marked arterial desaturation immediately following cardiopulmonary bypass. Greely et al.[84] have described how the clinical use of derived data facilitated pharmacologic management of intraoperative hypoxemic spells in a patient with tetralogy of Fallot. Figures 17-29 to 17-31 represent intraoperative delineation of a sinus venosus atrial septal defect, a membranous ventricular septal defect and anomalous origin of the coronary arteries, respectively. A representation of normal coronary architecture is presented in Figure 17-32.

Transesophageal imaging is likely to supplant epicardial analysis of the efficacy of valve repair and the detection of paraprosthetic peaks. It is ideally suited for differentiation between physiologic and pathologic flow across mitral prostheses (Figs. 17-33 and 17-34) and detection of paraprosthetic leaks. Transverse and longitudinal plane views of a vegetation emanating from the sewing ring of an aortic valve prosthesis are presented in Figure 17-35. Figure 17-36 represents a transverse plane view of an endocarditis-associated regurgitation of an aortic prosthesis. The abscess cavity was found to involve the interatrial septum. Figure 17-37 illustrates a transverse plane view of longstanding endocarditis of the mitral valve.

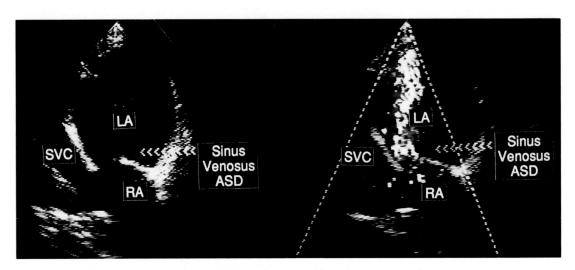

Fig. 17-29. Two-dimensional TEE and color Doppler longitudinal plane image of a sinus venosus atrial septal defect. LA, left atrium; RA, right atrium; SVC, superior vena cava.

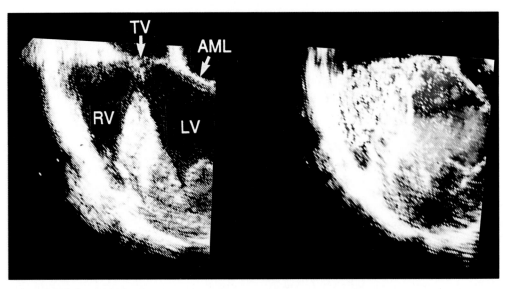

Fig. 17-30. Two-dimensional TEE and color Doppler transverse plane images of a membranous ventricula septal defect. AML, anterior mitral leaflet; LV, left ventricle; RV, right ventricle; TV, tricuspid valve.

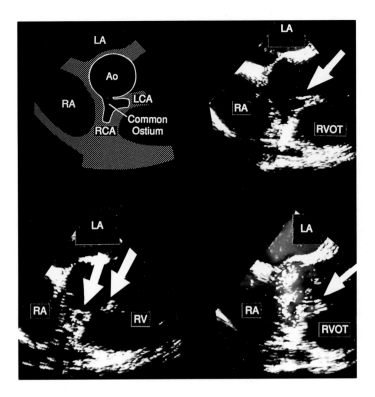

Fig. 17-31. Anomalous origin of the left coronary artery. *(Upper left)* Schematic representation depicting the right coronary artery (RCA), left main coronary artery (LCA) with a common ostium. *(Upper right)* Transesophageal transverse plane 2-D echocardiographic image depicting the origin of the LCA (arrow). *(Lower left)* Cross-sectional view of the RCA and LCA (arrows) slightly inferior to the previous image. *(Lower right)* Color Doppler image of flow within the ostium and LCA. Ao, aorta; LA, left atrium; RA, right atrium.

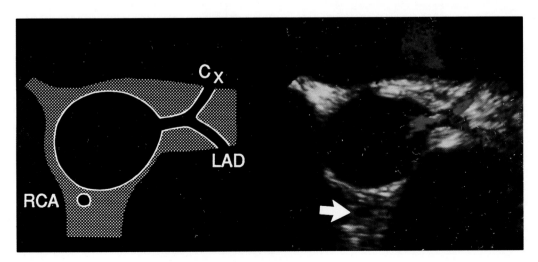

Fig. 17-32. Transverse plane 2-D TEE and color Doppler image of normal coronary arteries. Cx and LAD, circumflex and left anterior descending coronary arteries; RCA and arrow, right coronary artery; respectively.

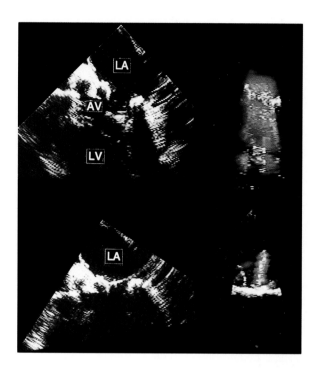

Fig. 17-33. Two-dimensional TEE and color Doppler image of a normally functioning nonbiologic mitral valve prosthesis. *(Upper left)* Transverse plane long-axis image of the St. Jude prosthesis during diastole. *(Upper right)* Corresponding color Doppler image, emphasizing the area of ultrasound "dropout." *(Lower left)* Image of the prosthesis during systole. *(Lower right)* Corresponding color Doppler image. The central and two lateral regurgitant jets *within* the sewing ring are normal findings. AV, aortic valve; LA, left atrium; LV, left ventricle.

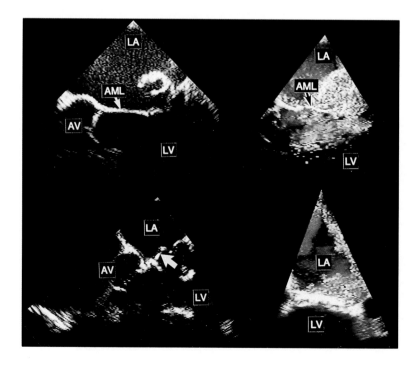

Fig. 17-34. Two-dimensional TEE and color Doppler transverse plane long-axis views of flail native and porcine mitral leaflets. *(Upper left)* Flail posterior mitral leaflet within the left atrium. Spontaneous echocardiographic contrast is present in the atrium. *(Upper right)* The resulting mitral regurgitant jet obscures the abnormal posterior leaflet. The anterior mitral leaflet is demarcated (arrow) for the purpose of orientation. *(Bottom left)* Flail leaflet of a porcine mitral valve (arrow). *(Bottom right)* The resulting mitral regurgitant jet can be seen to curve laterally and hug the wall of the left atrium. AV, aortic valve; AML, anterior mitral leaflet; LV, left ventricle.

Fig. 17-35. Two-dimensional TEE image of a vegetation within the ascending aorta obtained with a biplane probe. *(Top)* Transverse plane view of the vegetation (arrow). The proximal attachment was to the sewing ring of a prosthetic aortic valve. *(Bottom)* Longitudinal plane view of the vegetation (arrow). LA, left atrium; RPA, right pulmonary artery.

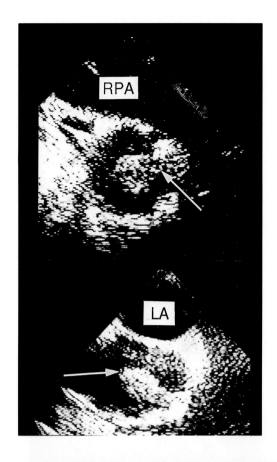

Fig. 17-36. Two-dimensional TEE and color Doppler transverse plane long-axis image of endocarditis originating in a nonbiologic aortic valvular prosthesis. *(Upper left)* Schematic representation illustrating the abscess and associated landmarks. *(Upper right)* Corresponding 2-D echocardiographic image illustrating the extent of the abscess. The anterior wedge-shaped area of ultrasound "dropout" is specific to the prosthesis. *(Bottom left)* Schematic representation illustrating the aortic regurgitant jet. *(Bottom right)* Corresponding color Doppler image illustrating the depth of penetration of the regurgitant jet. AML, anterior mitral leaflet; LA, left atrium; LV, left ventricle; RA, right atrium.

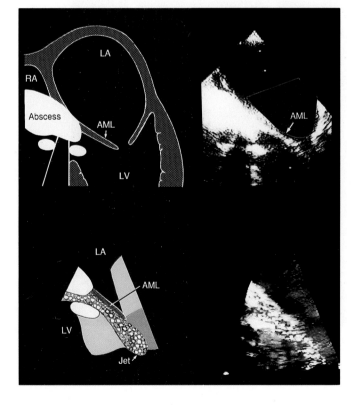

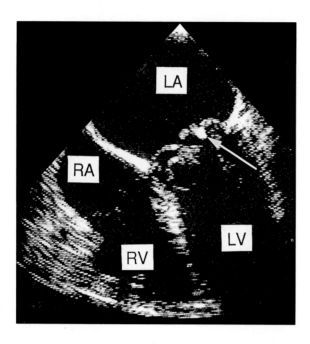

Fig. 17-37. Two-dimensional TEE transverse plane long-axis image of chronic endocarditis of the mitral valve. The calcification of the posterior leaflet (arrow) was associated with an underlying abscess cavity. LA, left atrium; LV, left ventricle; RA, right atrium; RV, right ventricle.

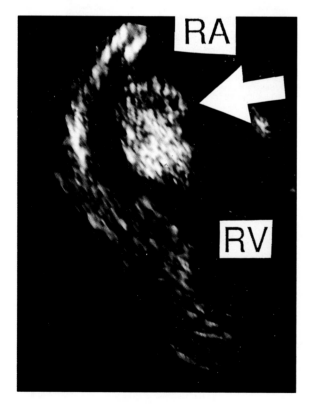

Fig. 17-38. Two-dimensional TEE transverse plane long-axis image of a right atrial thrombus. RA, right atrium; RV, right ventricle.

Fig. 17-39. Two-dimensional TEE transverse plane image of a right pulmonary artery embolus. *(Top)* Schematic representation of a transesophageal transverse plane image of a thrombus within the right pulmonary artery. *(Bottom)* Two-dimensional TEE image of the embolic thrombus (arrow). Ao, aorta; MPA, main pulmonary artery; RPA, right pulmonary artery; SVC, superior vena cava.

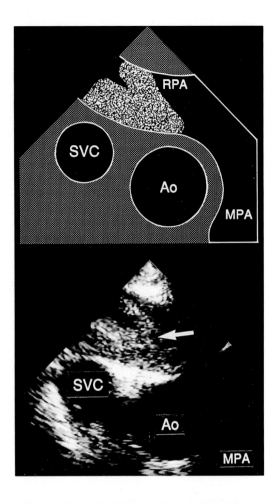

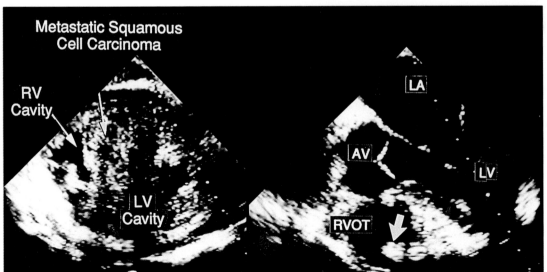

Fig. 17-40. Two-dimensional TEE transverse plane image of a metastatic squamous cell carcinoma. *(Left)* Transgastric short-axis view. The neoplasm involves the septum and posterior ventricular walls. *(Right)* Transesophageal long-axis view. The neoplasm (arrow) can be seen to extend to the right ventricular outflow tract. AV, aortic valve; LA, left atrium; LV, left ventricle; RV, right ventricle; RVOT, right ventricular outflow tract.

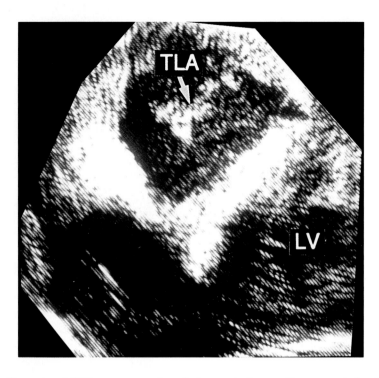

Fig. 17-41. Two-dimensional TEE transverse plane left ventricular papillary muscle level short-axis image depicting severe right ventricular volume overload. This patient presented with a right ventricular infarct and required support with a right heart assist device. LV, left ventricle; TLA, tricuspid leaflet apparatus.

Other intraoperative uses have also been described. Documentation exists for acute right heart dysfunction associated with a pulmonary embolism during liver transplantation,[85] embolization during insertion of hip prostheses.[86] Figures 17-38 and 17-39 illustrate a right atrial thrombus and a pulmonary artery embolus, respectively. Figure 17-40 demonstrates the use of intraoperative TEE to detail the extent of an intracardiac mass in a patient presenting for biopsy. The lesion subsequently defined as metastatic carcinoma, involved the septum and posterior wall of both ventricles, and extended superiorly to the right ventricular outflow tract. Figure 17-41 represents the echocardiographic findings in a patient with severe right heart dysfunction due to a right atrial and ventricular infarct.

A number of considerations pertain to internal mammary vein grafting cases. Adequate surgical exposure during "take-down" of the pedicle may necessitate that the underlying lung be allowed to become atelectatic. Transesophageal imaging can facilitate the assessment of the adequacy of reexpansion. When the pleura is breached, spillover of "topical cold" solution can occur during cardiopulmonary bypass, presenting as a pleural effusion (Fig. 17-42). A pericardial effusion is presented in Figure 17-43.

IMAGING IN CONJUNCTION WITH THE USE OF CARDIAC ASSIST DEVICES AND CARDIOPULMONARY BYPASS

The intra-aortic balloon pump can be readily defined by TEE (Fig. 17-44). This imaging technique has been

Fig. 17-42. Transesophageal transverse plane view of a pleural effusion. Ao, aorta.

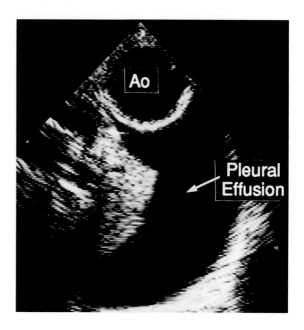

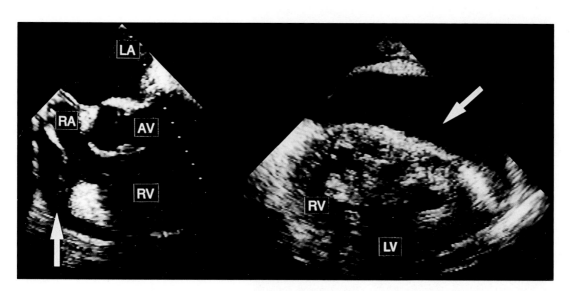

Fig. 17-43. Transesophageal transverse plane long-axis and short-axis views of a pericardial effusion (arrow). AV, aortic valve; LA, left atrium; LV, left ventricle; RA, right atrium; RV, right ventricle.

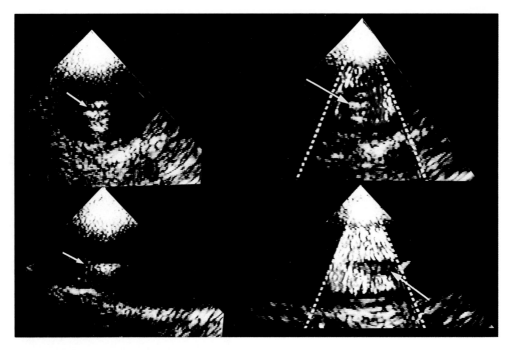

Fig. 17-44. Two-dimensional TEE and color Doppler images of an intra-aortic balloon pump using a biplane probe. These images were obtained during cardiopulmonary bypass when the intra-aortic balloon pump (arrow) was temporarily discontinued. The color Doppler patterns, consistent with turbulence, are associated with antegrade perfusion via the aortic root. *(Upper left)* Transverse plane image. *(Upper right)* Corresponding color Doppler image accentuating the outline of the device. *(Lower left)* Longitudinal plane image. *(Lower right)* Corresponding color Doppler image.

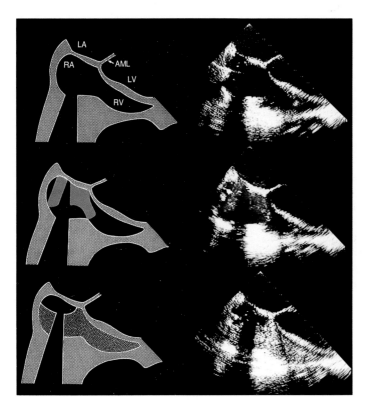

Fig. 17-45. Transesophageal transverse plane long-axis view of a right atrial two-stage single venous cannula. These images were obtained before cardiopulmonary bypass. *(Top)* Two-dimensional TEE image illustrating the ultrasound "drop-out" resulting from the presence of the cannula. *(Middle)* The superimposed color Doppler image highlights the above phenomenon. *(Bottom)* Saline-contrast echocardiographic delineation of the outline of the cannula. AML, anterior mitral leaflet; LA, left atrium; LV, left ventricle; RA, right atrium; RV, right ventricle.

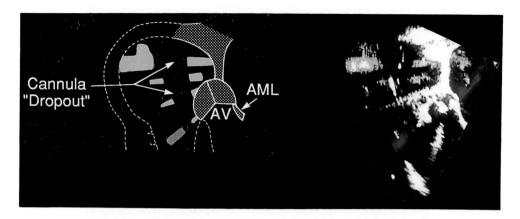

Fig. 17-46. Transesophageal transverse plane long-axis view of double venous cannulation of the right atrium. *(Left)* Schematic representation depicting ultrasound "dropout" within the right atrial cavity. *(Right)* Two-dimensional echocardiographic image with superimposed color Doppler mapping to accentuate the ultrasound-opaque characteristics of the cannulae. AML, anterior mitral leaflet; AV, aortic valve.

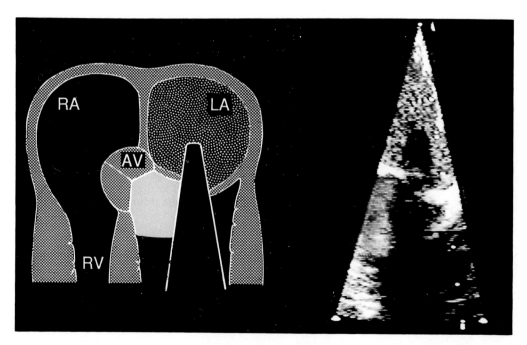

Fig. 17-47. Transesophageal transverse plane long-axis view of a pulmonary venous vent in the left atrium. *(Left)* Schematic representation of the associated ultrasound "drop-out." The aortic valve and right heart structures are shown for orientation purposes. *(Right)* A narrow window color Doppler image of the left atrium, anterior mitral leaflet, and proximal left ventricular outflow tract. The left atrium is also marked by spontaneous echocardiographic contrast. AV, aortic valve; LA, left atrium; RA, right atrium; RV, right ventricle.

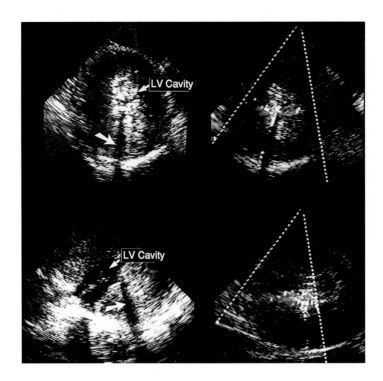

Fig. 17-48. Transgastric 2-D echocardiographic and color Doppler transverse and longitudinal plane images of a left ventricular apical drainage vent using a biplane probe. These images were obtained during total cardiopulmonary bypass. *(Upper left)* Two-dimensional echocardiographic transverse plane short-axis view illustrating the ultrasound "dropout" (arrow) caused by the cannula. The left ventricular cavity is essentially obliterated. *(Upper right)* The color Doppler image helps define the left ventricular cavity margins. *(Lower left)* Corresponding 2-D echocardiographic longitudinal plane view of the ventricle. The arrow indicates the ultrasound "dropout." *(Lower right)* The corresponding color Doppler image.

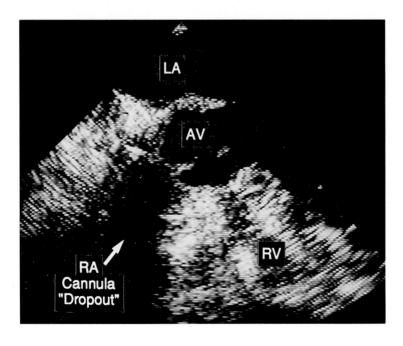

Fig. 17-49. Two-dimensional TEE transverse plane long-axis image depicting cardiopulmonary bypass associated right heart decompression. The right atrial (RA) single venous cannula is associated with image "dropout." The right ventricle (RV) is totally obliterated. AV, aortic valve; LA, left atrium.

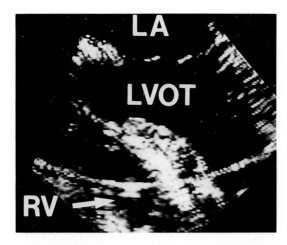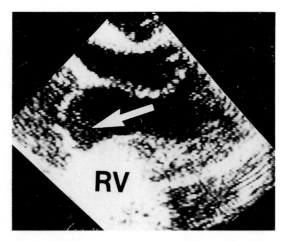

Fig. 17-50. Two-dimensional TEE transverse plane long-axis image representing cardiopulmonary bypass associated total decompression of the right ventricle. *(Left)* Transverse plane 2-D TEE image depicting the right ventricle (RV), left ventricular outflow tract (LVOT), and left atrium (LA). *(Right)* The RV can be seen to be totally cavity obliterated. The LA decompression, associated in this case with venting, is morphologically apparent by the infolding of the posterior wall. Cavitations, associated with administration of crystalloid cardioplegia, can be seen within the LVOT (arrow). The right heart catheter in both panels presents with a split-image artifact. (From Rafferty et al.,[66] with permission.)

used to facilitate optimal positioning of the device. The use of left ventricular, right ventricular, and biventricular assist devices and institution of conventional partial and total cardiopulmonary bypass are also associated with placement of intravascular cannulae. These ultrasound-opaque prostheses can impede imaging, as illustrated in Figures 17-45 to 17-48, representing right atrial and pulmonary vein drainage cannulae and left ventricular apical vents, respectively. In addition, the unique extremes of cardiac decompression associated with cardiopulmonary bypass can alter the morphology and orientation of characteristic landmark structures, making orientation difficult, particularly under conditions of asystole (Figs. 17-49 and 17-50).

DETECTION OF AIR EMBOLI

In certain neurosurgical procedures and all cardiac procedures, the prevention, early detection, and treatment of air emboli are cornerstones of management.[87-91] Intraoperative TEE represents the most sensitive available monitor of intravascular air and is routinely employed as a guide to such prophylaxis and therapy at many institutions. A clinical presentation of intracardiac air associated with a mitral valve repair and annuloplasty is illustrated in Figure 17-51. Air caused by pulmonary venous vent placement (Fig. 17-52) can be distinguished from other causes by analysis of its origin and timing.

DEFINITION OF THE POTENTIAL FOR ATHEROMATOUS EMBOLIC PHENOMENA

The value of TEE in the diagnosis of aortic dissection is well established.[92-98] The incidence of unsuspected severe aortic atheromatous disease in patients re-

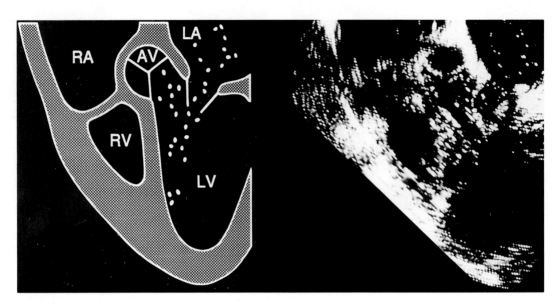

Fig. 17-51. Two-dimensional TEE transverse plane long-axis image depicting intracardiac air associated with mitral valve repair and annuloplasty. AV, aortic valve; LA, left atrium; LV, left ventricle; RA, right atrium; RV, right ventricle.

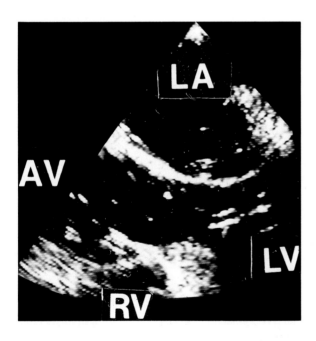

Fig. 17-52. Intracardiac cavitations associated with insertion of a vent into the right upper pulmonary vein. The vent has not yet been advanced into the left atrium. The cavitations can be distinguished from other causes of intracardiac air by analysis of their origin and timing. AV, aortic valve; LA, left atrium; LV, left ventricle; RV, right ventricle.

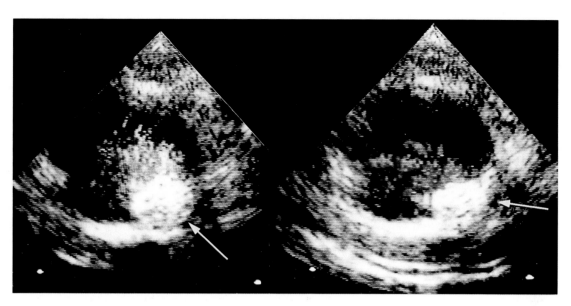

Fig. 17-53. Two-dimensional TEE transverse plane images of the descending thoracic aorta illustrating atheromatous plaques protruding into the lumen. The posterior margins of the lesions are highlighted by color Doppler coding.

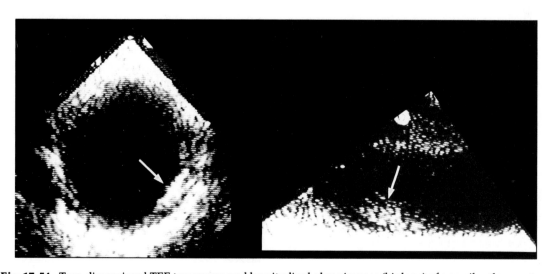

Fig. 17-54. Two-dimensional TEE transverse and longitudinal plane images (biplane) of a sessile atheromatous plaque in the descending thoracic aorta.

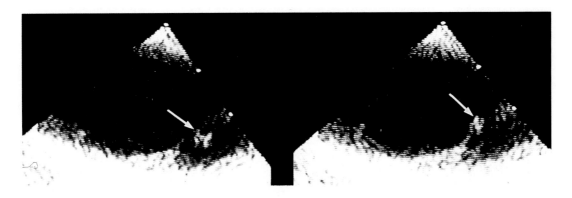

Fig. 17-55. Two-dimensional TEE longitudinal plane images of a pedunculated atheromatous plaque in the descending thoracic aorta. The sequential frames illustrate the mobility of the lesion.

ferred for other diagnoses has been reported to be as high as 25 percent.[99] It is becoming increasingly recognized that the aorta represents a potential site of origin for embolic material that might be dislodged during manipulation and cannulation of the aorta. A combination of transverse and longitudinal views permits sequential evaluation of the aortic arch, transverse and descending aorta. A variety of descending thoracic aorta images are presented in Figures 17-53 to 17-55.

CONTRAST ECHOCARDIOGRAPHY

Rapid intravascular administration of crystalloid is associated with agitation of the infused solution. The resulting cavitation (microbubble) formation provides an ultrasound-opaque medium that can be used as a source of contrast[100,101] (Figs. 17-56 and 17-57). Saline-contrast echocardiography, with agitation of saline by preinjection ballottement, is an established echocardiography imaging technique that has been applied to quantification of right ventricular function, diagnosis of intracardiac shunting, assessment of aortic, mitral and tricuspid valve integrity, definition of myocardial flow distribution, and localization of intravascular catheters.[102-112] The analogous use of antegrade crystalloid cardioplegia as an imaging agent is presented in Figures 17-58 and 17-59. The use of this technique in the transesophageal diagnosis of an incidental atrial septal defect in a CABG patient is illustrated in Figures 17-60 to 17-62.

The technique has also been variously refined by combining saline with specific contrast agents[113-117] and stabilizing compounds.[118-122] More recently, sonication of such contrast solutions has been shown to produce uniformly sized cavitations[123-126] with diameters of small enough caliber to pass through capillaries.[127,128] These sonicated solutions have been investigated to assess their ability to demarcate regional

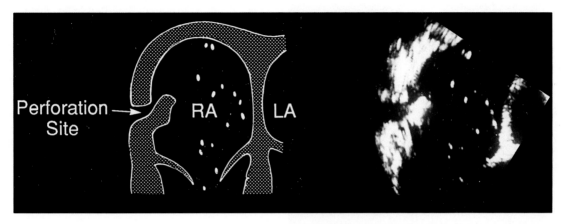

Fig. 17-56. Two-dimensional TEE transverse plane image of right atrial cavitations associated with infusion of resuscitative fluids in a patient with a right atrial perforation. LA, left atrium; RA, right atrium.

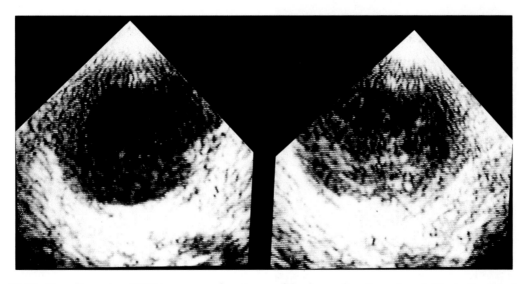

Fig. 17-57. Two-dimensional TEE transverse plane image of the descending thoracic aorta illustrating intraluminal cavitations associated with infusion of a bolus of crystalloid prime via an aortic arch cannula. *(Left)* Initiation of the infusion. *(Right)* Peak of the infusion.

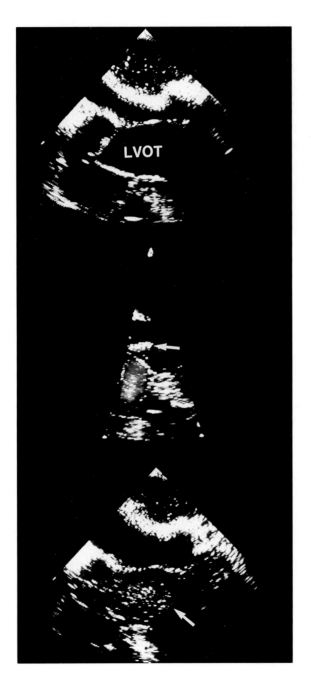

Fig. 17-58. Transesophageal transverse plane 2-D echocardiographic image of antegrade crystalloid cardioplegia in a patient with pre-existing aortic regurgitation. *(Top)* Left ventricular outflow tract (LVOT) during cardiopulmonary bypass. Associated cardiac decompression has caused infolding of the left atrial (LA) wall, causing it to appear thickened. Extracardiac posteriorly located cavitations are due to "topical cold" solution. *(Middle)* Color Doppler representation of the pre-existing aortic regurgitant jet (arrow). *(Bottom)* Cardioplegia regurgitation, as evidenced by cavitations within the LVOT. (From Rafferty et al.,[66] with permission.)

Fig. 17-59. Transgastric transverse plane 2-D echocardiographic image of regurgitant antegrade crystalloid cardioplegia within the body of the left ventricle. LV, left ventricle; RV, right ventricle.

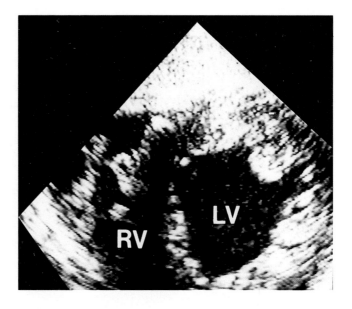

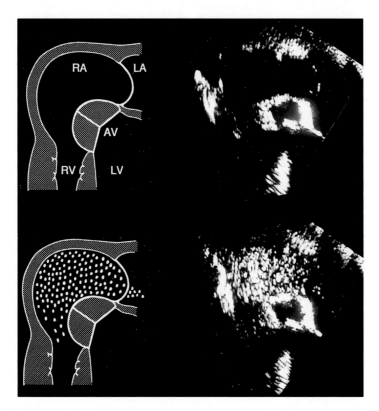

Fig. 17-60. Bidirectional ostium secundum atrial septal defect. Saline-contrast diagnosis of right-to-left shunt. *(Top)* Representation of right to left pressure gradient evidenced by bowing of the septum to the left. *(Bottom)* Transseptal passage of saline contrast.

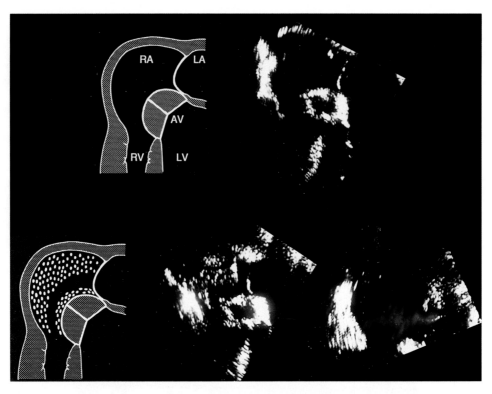

Fig. 17-61. Bidirectional ostium secundum atrial septal defect. Negative saline-contrast diagnosis of left-to-right shunt. *(Top)* Representation of left-to-right pressure gradient evidenced by bowing of the septum to the right. *(Lower right and middle)* Left atrial blood containing minimal contrast has displaced the contrast-containing blood in the right atrium. *(Lower left)* The area of ''negative'' contrast in the middle panel corresponds to the color Doppler left-to-right shunt flow.

myocardial perfusion differences at arteriography,[129] during angioplasty,[130] and both during and after cardiopulmonary bypass.[131,132]

SPONTANEOUS ECHOCARDIOGRAPHIC CONTRAST

The phenomenon whereby swirling smokelike patterns occur in the cardiac chambers or great vessels in the absence of intravascular injection is known as spontaneous echocardiographic contrast. This opacification is usually associated with stagnant blood flow[133–137] and is believed to be caused by red blood cell aggregation.[138–140] Platelet aggregation has also been implicated as a possible cause by one group of investigators.[141,142] The left atrium represents the most common site for this entity, frequent associations being atrial fibrillation, increased left atrial dimensions, prosthetic mitral valves, and mitral stenosis. However, the phenomenon has been observed in both sides of the heart, as well as in the great vessels.[143–148] In one series, spontaneous echocardiographic contrast was a predictor of the presence of left atrial thrombus and systemic embolization.[149] The most frequent associations in the left ventricle are poor contractility, either global or regional, and the presence of an aneurysm, respectively. Figures 17-63 and 17-64 represent an example of spontaneous contrast in a descending thoracic aneurysm.

Fig. 17-62. Bidirectional ostium secundum atrial septal defect. Equalization of right and left atrial pressures. *(Top)* The interatrial septum can be seen to have assumed a midline position, reflecting the absence of a gradient. *(Bottom)* Saline-contrast imaging does not depict the septal defect, emphasizing the importance of considering the interatrial pressure gradient to avoid false-negative diagnoses.

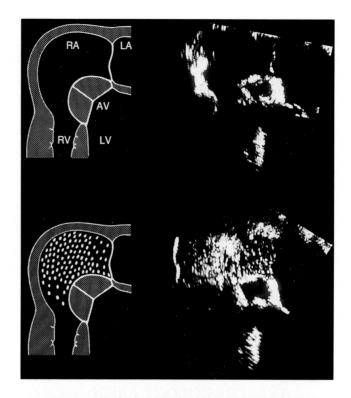

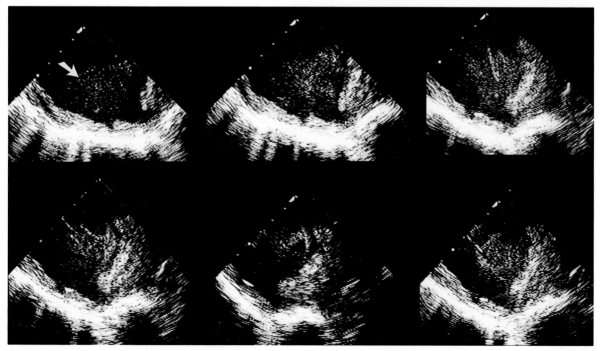

Fig. 17-63. Spontaneous echocardiographic contrast. Sequential frames of transesophageal transverse plane images of a descending thoracic aneurysm illustrating the swirling pattern of echocardiographic "smoke" (arrow).

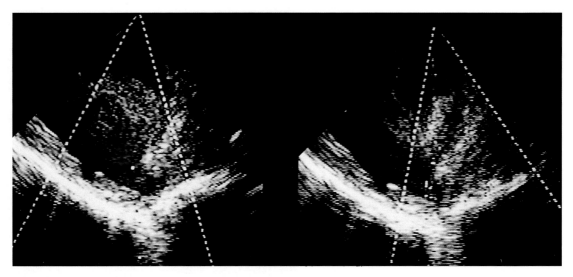

Fig. 17-64. Color Doppler image of the spontaneous echocardiographic contrast depicted in Figure 17-62.

QUALITY ASSURANCE IN ANESTHESIOLOGY-BASED INTRAOPERATIVE ECHOCARDIOGRAPHY MONITORING PROGRAMS

The establishment of a quality assurance system is essential for the credibility and structured growth of anesthesiology-based transesophageal echocardiography programs. Guidelines of the Yale-New Haven Hospital Department of Anesthesiology program include the following:

1. Hospital and anesthesia record documentation of transesophageal examinations
2. Completion of an examination database form
3. Provision of a videocassette recording for each case, for subsequent formal evaluation and grading by dedicated ultrasonographers
4. Storage of the videocassette recordings in an archival filing system
5. Technician maintenance of a daily log of personnel responsible for endoscope requisition
6. Data entry into a permanent computer database, with notation of lesions suitable for educational and research purposes
7. Scheduled conferences featuring review of contemporaneous cases
8. Continuing medical education and basic imaging principles

A recently presented evaluation of 846 consecutive cases in our program[150] demonstrated that resources were directed primarily to the adult cardiac surgery service. This distribution of cases should not be construed as an ultimate goal. Rather, it would be hoped that the application of transesophageal endoscopy would reflect general operative risk, recognizing that such monitoring must take precedence in certain specific instances, such as valve repair. However, redistribution should not occur other than in tandem with maintenance of minimum quality assurance standards by involved personnel, who may or may not have had extensive echocardiography experience. The acquisition of the appropriate skills requires considerable dedication in terms of time and effort, for which there is no substitute. Future department policy will require an objectively demonstrated level of commitment for endoscope requisition requests to be honored.

Adverse sequelae in our series consisted of a chipped tooth, a transient unilateral vocal cord paresis, and ingestion of glutaraldehyde disinfectant solution, respectively. The vocal cord paresis resolved spontaneously within 3 months and may have been caused by prolonged intubation. The ingestion of glutaraldehyde disinfectant solution was associated with a defect in the endoscope outer sheath, with endoscope

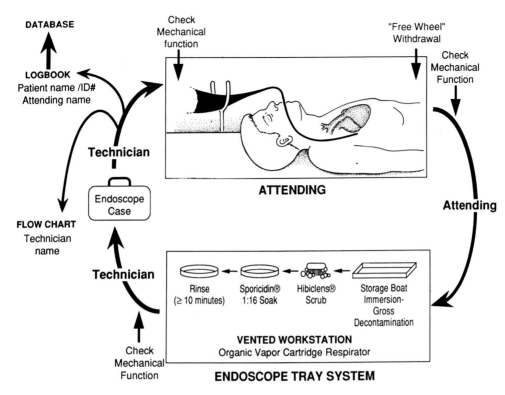

Fig. 17-65. Endoscope requisition cycle illustrating the evidentiary chain allocating primary responsibility.

placement being associated with retrograde discharge of sequestered disinfectant.

Surprisingly, equipment mishaps represented a major problem. Console mishaps consisted of avulsion of an ECG cable and dislocation of an outer side panel, respectively. Loss of the integrity of the endoscope outer sheath occurred on two further occasions, being associated with a clean linear slit and a tooth mark, respectively. The former was assumed to be malicious in origin, and the latter from failure to employ the appropriate mouth guard. Near-mishaps consisted of abandonment of the endoscope in the operating room at procedure conclusion on four occasions. Because these misadventures were thought to be related to lack of due care, we have instituted an evidentiary chain whereby endoscopes are tracked sequentially throughout use. Release of the instrument from a central storage area initiates documentation identifying responsible personnel throughout the requisition cycle (Fig. 17-65).

REFERENCES

1. Tennant R, Wiggers C. The effect of coronary occlusion on myocardial contraction. Am J Physiol 1935; 112:351.
2. Smith J, Cahalan M, Benefiel D, et al. Intraoperative detection of myocardial ischemia in high risk patients: electrocardiography versus two-dimensional transesophageal echocardiography. Circulation 1985; 72:1015.
3. Clements F, DeBruijn N. Perioperative evaluation of regional wall motion by transesophageal two-dimensional echocardiography. Anesth Analg 1987; 6:249.
4. Wohlgelernter D, Jaffe C, Cabin H, et al. Silent ischemia during coronary occlusion produced by balloon inflation: relation to regional myocardial dysfunction. J Am Coll Cardiol 1987; 10:491.
5. Hauser A, Gangadharan V, Ramos R, et al. Sequence of mechanical, electrocardiographic and clinical effects of repeated coronary artery occlusion in human beings: echocardiographic observations during coronary angioplasty. J Am Coll Cardiol 1985; 5:193.
6. Wohlgelernter D, Cleman M, Highman H, et al. Regional myocardial dysfunction during coronary angioplasty: evaluation by two-dimensional echocardiography and 12 lead electrocardiography. J Am Coll Cardiol 1986; 7:1245.
7. Leung J, O'Kelley B, Browner W, et al. Prognostic importance of postbypass regional wall motion abnormalities in patients undergoing coronary artery bypass graft surgery. Anesthesiology 1989; 71:16.

8. Harris S, Gordon M, Urban M, et al. The pressure rate quotient is not an indicator of myocardial ischemia in humans — an echocardiographic evaluation. Anesthesiology 1990; 73:A157.

9. London M, Tubau J, Wong M. The natural history of segmental wall motion abnormalities in patients undergoing noncardiac surgery. Anesthesiology 1990; 73:644.

10. Schluter M, Langenstein B, Popster J, et al. Transesophageal cross-sectional echocardiography with a phased array transducer system. Technique and initial clinical results. Br Heart J 1982; 48:67.

11. Schluter M, Hinrichs A, Thier W, et al. Transesophageal two-dimensional echocardiography: comparison of ultrasonic and anatomic sections. Am J Cardiol 1984; 53:1173.

12. Seward J, Khandheria B, Oh J, et al. Transesophageal echocardiography: technique, anatomic correlations, implementation, and clinical applications. Mayo Clin Proc 1988; 63:649.

13. Abel M, Nishimura R, Callahan M, et al. Evaluation of intraoperative transesophageal two-dimensional echocardiography. Anesthesiology 1987; 66:64.

14. Konstadt S, Thys D, Mindich B, et al. Validation of quantitative intraoperative transesophageal echocardiography. Anesthesiology 1986; 65:418.

15. Seward J, Khandheria B, Edwards W, et al. Biplanar transesophageal echocardiography: anatomic correlations, image orientation and clinical applications. Mayo Clin Proc 1990; 65:1193.

16. Matsuzaki M, Toma Y, Kusukawa R. Clinical applications of transesophageal echocardiography. Circulation 1990; 82:709.

17. Panadian N, Skorton D, Collins S, et al. Heterogeneity of left ventricular segmental wall thickening and excursion in two-dimensional echocardiograms of normal human subjects. Am J Cardiol 1983; 51:1667.

18. Lehmann K, Lee F, McKenzie W, et al. Onset of altered interventricular septal motion during cardiac surgery — assessment by continuous intraoperative echocardiography. Circulation 1990; 82:1325.

19. Stamm R, Carabello B, Mayers D, Martin R. Two-dimensional echocardiographic measurement of left ventricular ejection fraction: prospective analysis of what constitutes an adequate determination. Am Heart J 1982; 104:136.

20. Clements F, Harpole D, Quill T, et al. Estimation of left ventricular volume and ejection fraction by two-dimensional transoesophageal echocardiography: comparison of short axis imaging and simultaneous angiography. Br J Anaesth 1990; 64:331.

21. Urbanowitz J, Shaabon J, Cohen N, et al. Comparison of transesophageal echocardiographic and scintigraphic estimates of left ventricular end-diastolic volume index and ejection fraction in patients following coronary artery bypass grafting. Anesthesiology 1990; 72:607.

22. Cahalan M, Ionescu P, Melton H. Automated real-time analysis of transesophageal echocardiograms. Anesthesiology 1991; 75:A385.

23. Waggoner A, Perez J, Barzilai B, et al. Real-time two-dimensional derived left ventricular (LV) diastolic and systolic areas and fractional area change using automatic boundary detection. J Am Soc Echocardiogr 1991; 4:304.

24. Perez J, Waggoner A, Thomas L, et al. Real-time quantitation of left ventricular (LV) areas during dobutamine stress echocardiography. J Am Soc Echocardiogr 1991; 4:280.

25. Vandenberg B, Rath L, Stuhmuller P, et al. Estimation of left ventricular cavity area with a new, on-line automated echocardiographic edge detection system. J Am Coll Cardiol 1991; 17:291A.

26. Perez J, Waggoner A, Barzilai B, et al. New edge detection algorithm facilitates two-dimensional echocardiographic on-line analysis of left ventricular (LV) performance. J Am Coll Cardiol 1991; 17:291A.

27. Klein S, Waggoner A, Holland J, et al. Echocardiographic on-line measurement and display of left ventricular (LV) cavity areas and function: reproducibility and normal values in control subjects. Circulation 1991; 84:II-584.

28. Scharma M, Kieso R, Fleagle S, et al. Real-time, on-line echocardiographic measurement of LV function using an automated border detection system. Circulation 1991; 84:II-585.

29. Iliceto S, Pellegrini C, Napoli F, et al. Automatic evaluation of stress induced left ventricular area changes with a new on-line echocardiographic edge detection system. Circulation 1991; 84:II-585.

30. Durkin M, Rafferty T. TAPSE can be reproducibly quantified by transesophageal echocardiography. Anesthesiology 1990; 73:A468.

31. Kaul S, Tei C, Hopkins J, Shah P. Assessment of right ventricular function using two-dimensional echocardiography. Am Heart J 1984; 107:526.

32. Hammarstrom E, Wranne B, Pinto F, et al. Tricuspid annular motion. J Am Soc Echo 1991; 4:131.

33. Feigenbaum H: Echocardiography. Philadelphia: Lea & Febiger, 1986.

34. Rafferty T, Durkin M, Elefteriades J, et al. Right ventricular wall motion following cardiopulmonary bypass. Anesthesiology 1990; 73:A158.

35. Rafferty T, Durkin M, Harris S, et al. Transesophageal two-dimensional echocardiographic analysis of right ventricular systolic performance indices during coronary artery bypass graft surgery. J Cardiothorac Vasc Anesth (in press).

36. Bommer W, Weinert L, Neumann A, et al. Determination of right atrial and right ventricular size by two-dimensional echocardiography. Circulation 1979; 60:91.

37. Durkin M, Rafferty T. Two-dimensional echocardiographic determination of right ventricular maximum minor axis fractional shortening. Anesthesiology 1990; 73:A542.

38. Jardin F, Gueret P, Dubourg O, et al. Right ventricular volumes by thermodilution in the adult respiratory distress syndrome: a comparative study using two-dimensional echocardiography as a reference. Chest 1985; 88:34.

39. Jardin F, Brun-Ney D, Hardy A, et al. Combined thermodilution and two-dimensional echocardiographic evaluation of right ventricular function during respiratory support with PEEP. Chest 1991; 99:162.

40. Koorn R, Reich D, Tamman R, et al. Right ventricular ejection fraction measurement: thermodilution versus 2-D transesophageal echocardiography. Anesthesiology 1991; 75:A386.

41. Maurer G, Nanda N: Two-dimensional echocardiographic evaluation of exercise-induced left and right ventricular asynergy: correlation with thallium scanning. Am J Cardiol 1981; 48:720.

42. Ohman M, Helmy S, Stern H, et al. In vitro relationship of jet flow area by Doppler color flow: Are there correlations? J Am Coll Cardiol 1988; 11:19A.

43. Thomas J, Davidoff R, Wilkins G, et al. The volume of a color flow jet varies directly with flow rate and inversely with orifice size: a hydrodynamic in vitro assessment. J Am Coll Cardiol 1988; 11:19A.

44. Davidoff R, Wilkins G, Thomas J, et al. Regurgitant volumes by color flow overestimates injected volumes in an in vitro model. J Am Coll Cardiol 1987; 9:110A.

45. Ofili E, Kouchoukos N, Wareing T: Transesophageal echocardiographic determinants of prognosis in ischemic mitral regurgitation. J Am Soc Echo 1991; 4:298.

46. Tamura T, Krabill K, Sahn D. Determinants of spatial resolution of color flow Doppler imaging systems: in vitro investigation. J Am Coll Cardiol 1987; 9:111A.

47. Sahn D, Valdes-Cruz L, Swensson E, et al. Potential for angular errors in Doppler gradient estimates: a study of spatial orientation of jet lesions using real-time color flow-Doppler imaging. Circulation 1984; 70(suppl II):115.

48. Ashrafzadeh A, Dormer K, Cheung J. A two-dimensional ultrasonic probe for flow measurement. Biomed Instrum Tech 1989; 23:301.

49. Tamura T, Yoganalhan A, Sohn D. In vitro methods for studying the accuracy of velocity determination and spatial resolution of a color Doppler flow mapping system. Am Heart J 1987; 114:152.

50. Miyatake K, Izumi S, Okamoto M, et al. Semi-quantitative grading of severity of mitral regurgitation by real-time two-dimensional Doppler flow imaging technique. J Am Coll Cardiol 1986; 1:82.

51. Maurer G, Czer L, Chaux A, et al. Intraoperative Doppler color flow mapping for assessment of valve repair for mitral regurgitation. Am J Cardiol 1987; 60:333.

52. Czer L, Maurer G, Bolger A, et al. Intraoperative evaluation of mitral regurgitation by Doppler color flow mapping. Circulation 1987; 76(suppl III):108.

53. Reichert S, Visser C, Moulijn A, et al. Intraoperative transesophageal color-coded Doppler echocardiography for evaluation of residual regurgitation after mitral valve repair. J Thorac Cardiovasc Surg 1990; 100:756.

54. Mohr-Kahaly S, Erbel R, Zenker G, et al. Semi-quantitative grading of mitral regurgitation by color-coded Doppler echocardiography. Int J Cardiol 1989; 23:223.

55. Spain M, Smith M, Grayburn P, et al. Quantitative assessment of mitral regurgitation by Doppler color flow imaging: angiographic and hemodynamic correlations. J Am Coll Cardiol 1989; 13:585.

56. Nellessen U, Schnittger I, Appleton C, et al. Transesophageal two-dimensional echocardiography and color Doppler flow velocity mapping in the evaluation of cardiac valve prostheses. Circulation 1988; 78:848.

57. Helmcke F, Nanda N, Hsiung M, et al. Color Doppler assessment of mitral regurgitation with orthogonal planes. Circulation 1987; 75:175.

58. Sahn D: Instrumentation and physical factors related to visualization of stenotic and regurgitant jets by Doppler color flow mapping. J Am Coll Cardiol 1988; 12:1354.

59. Krabill K, Tamura T, Sahn D, et al. The shape of regurgitant jets: in vitro flow visualization and color flow Doppler studies. J Am Coll Cardiol 1987; 9:110A.

60. Liu M, Louie E. Independent pulsed Doppler mapping techniques. Limitations in the prediction of the angiographic severity of mitral regurgitation. Chest 1989; 96:1263.

61. Carter J, Davis E. Comparison of mitral valve regurgitant jet areas by biplane transesophageal echocardiography. Anesthesiology 1991; 75:A389.

62. Wong M, Matsumura M, Suzuki K, Omoto R. Technical and biologic sources of variability in the mapping of aortic, mitral and tricuspid color flow jets. Am J Cardiol 1987; 60:847.

63. Akasaka T, Yoshikawa J, Yoshida K, et al. Age related valvular regurgitation: a study by pulsed Doppler echocardiography. Circulation 1987; 76:262.

64. Meyerowitz C, Jacobs L, Wertheimer J, et al. Assessment of aortic regurgitation by transesophageal echocardiography — correlation with angiographic determination. J Am Soc Echo 1991; 4:278.

65. Davis E, Rafferty T, Durkin M, et al. Transesophageal color flow-Doppler imaging of aortic insufficiency in cardiac surgery patients. J Am Soc Echo 1991; 4:289.

66. Rafferty T, Durkin M, Sittig D, et al. Transesophageal color flow-Doppler imaging of aortic insufficiency in cardiac surgery patients. J Thorac Cardiovasc Surg 104:521, 1992.

67. Miyatake K, Okamoto M, Kinoshita N, et al. Clinical applications of a new type of real-time two-dimensional Doppler flow imaging system. Am J Cardiol 1984; 54:857.

68. Omoto R, Yokote Y, Takamoto S, et al. The development of real-time two-dimensional Doppler echocardiography and its clinical significance in acquired valvular diseases. Jpn Heart J 1984; 25:325.

69. Perry G, Helmcke F, Nanda N, et al. Evaluation of aortic insufficiency by Doppler color flow mapping. J Am Coll Cardiol 1987; 9:952.

70. Switzer D, Yoganathan A, Nanda N, et al. Calibration of color Doppler flow mapping during extreme hemodynamic conditions in vitro: a foundation for a reliable quantitative grading system for aortic incompetence. Circulation 1987; 75:837.

71. Miyatake K, Okamoto M, Kinoshita N, et al. Evaluation of tricuspid regurgitation by pulsed Doppler and two-dimensional echocardiography. Circulation 1982; 66:777.

72. Kostucki W, Vandengossche J-L, Friart A, Englert M. Pulsed Doppler regurgitant flow patterns of normal valves. Am J Cardiol 1986; 58:309.

73. Yoshida K, Yoshikawa J, Shakudo M, et al. Color Doppler evaluation of valvular regurgitation in normal subjects. Circulation 1988; 78:840.

74. Rafferty T, Durkin M, Matthew J. Estimation of tricuspid regurgitation: color flow Doppler versus saline-contrast echocardiography. Anesth Analg 1991; 72:S219.

75. Rafferty T, Durkin M, Harris S, et al. Color flow-Doppler tricuspid regurgitation should be expressed as a function of right atrial dimensions. J Clin Monit 1992; 7:A-S214.

76. Takamoto S, Kyo S, Adachi H, et al. Intraoperative color flow mapping by real-time two-dimensional Doppler echocardiography for evaluation of valvular and congenital heart disease and vascular disease. J Thorac Cardiovasc Surg 1985; 90:802.

77. Sutherland G, Fraser A. Color flow mapping in cardiology: indications and limitations. Br Med Bull 1989; 45:1076.

78. Hagler D, Tajiik A, Seward J, et al. Intraoperative two-dimensional Doppler echocardiography. A preliminary study for congenital heart disease. J Thorac Cardiovasc Surg 1988; 95:516.

79. Cyran S, Kimball T, Meyer R, et al. Efficacy of intraoperative transesophageal echocardiography in children with congenital heart disease. Am J Cardiol 1989; 63:594.

80. Kyo S, Omoto R, Matsumura M, et al. Intraoperative transesophageal echocardiography in pediatric patients. J Thorac Cardiovasc Surg 1990; 99:373.

81. Kyo S, Koike K, Takanawa E, et al. Impact of transesophageal Doppler echocardiography on pediatric cardiac surgery. Int J Cardiac Imag 1989; 4:41.

82. Kyo S, Takamoto S, Matsumura M, et al. Immediate and early postoperative evaluation of results of cardiac surgery by transesophageal two-dimensional Doppler echocardiography. Circulation 1987; 76:V113.

83. Dan M, Bonato R, Mazzucco A, et al: Value of transesophageal echocardiography during repair of congenital heart defects. Ann Thorac Surg 50:637, 1990.

84. Greeley W, Stanley T, Ungerleider R, et al: Intraoperative hypoxemic spells in Tetralogy of Fallot: an echocardiographic analysis of diagnosis and treatment. Anesth Analg 1989; 68:815.

85. Ellis J, Lichtor J, Feinstein S, et al. Right heart dysfunction, pulmonary embolism and paradoxical embolization during liver transplantation: a transesophageal two-dimensional echocardiographic study. Anesth Analg 1989; 68:777.

86. Ulrich C, Burri C, Worsdorfer O, Heinrich H. Intraoperative transesophageal two-dimensional echocardiography in total hip replacement. Arch Orthop Trauma Surg 1986; 105:274.

87. Cucchiara R, Nugent M, Seward J, et al. Air embolism in upright neurosurgical patients: detection and localization by two-dimensional transesophageal echocardiography. Anesthesiology 1984; 60:325.

88. Oka Y, Moriwaki K, Hong Y, et al. Detection of air emboli in the left heart by M-mode transesophageal echocardiography following cardiopulmonary bypass. Anesthesiology 1985; 63:109.

89. Oka Y, Inoue T, Hong Y, et al. Retained intracardiac air: transesophageal echocardiography for definition of incidence and monitoring removal by improved techniques. J Thorac Cardiovasc Surg 1986; 91:329.

90. Topol E, Humphrey L, Borkon A, et al. Value of intraoperative left ventricular microbubbles detected by transesophageal two-dimensional echocardiography in predicting neurologic outcome after cardiac operations. Am J Cardiol 1985; 56:773.

91. Calalang C, Shapiro J, Schwartz K, et al. Assessment of microembolization during cardiopulmonary bypass by transesophageal echocardiography. Anesthesiology 1991; 75:A64.

92. Iliceto S, Nanda N, Rizzon P, et al. Color Doppler evaluation of aortic dissection. Circulation 1987; 76:748.

93. Takamoto S, Omoto R. Visualization of thoracic dissecting aortic aneurysm by transesophageal Doppler color flow mapping. Hertz 1987; 12:187.

94. Borner N, Erbel R, Braun B, et al. Diagnosis of aortic dissection by transesophageal echocardiography. Am J Cardiol 1984; 54:1157.

95. DeBruijn N, Clements F, Kisslo J. Transesophageal applications of color flow imaging. Echocardiography 1987; 4:557.

96. Goldman M, Guarino T, Mindich B. Localization of aortic dissection intimal flap by intraoperative two-dimensional echocardiography. J Am Coll Cardiol 1985; 6:1155.

97. Erbel R, Daniel W, Vissen C, et al. Echocardiography and diagnosis of aortic dissection. A multicenter cooperative study. Lancet 1989; 1:457.

98. Mugge A, Daniel W, Laas J, et al. False negative diagnosis of proximal aortic dissection by computed tomography or angiography and possible explanations based on transesophageal echocardiographic findings. Am J Cardiol 1989; 64:1168.

99. Lanza G, Zabalgorita-Reyes M, Frazin L, et al. Plaque and structural characteristics of the descending thoracic aorta using transesophageal echocardiography. J Am Soc Echo 1991; 4:19.

100. Kremkau E, Gramiak R, Cartenson E. Ultrasonic detection of cavitation at catheter tips. AJR 1970; 110:177.

101. Meltzer R, Tickner E, Sahines T, Popp R. The source of ultrasonic contrast. JCU 1980; 8:121.

102. Wann S, Stickels K, Virindergit B, Gross C. Digital processing of contrast echocardiograms: a new technique for measuring right ventricular ejection fraction. Am J Cardiol 1984; 53:1164.

103. Fraker T, Harris P, Behar V, Kisslo J. Detection and exclusion of interatrial shunts by two-dimensional echocardiography and peripheral venous injection. Circulation 1979; 59:379.

104. Konstadt S, Louie E, Black S, et al. Intraoperative detection of patent foramen ovale by transesophageal echocardiography. Anesthesiology 1991; 74:212.

105. Gramiak R, Shah P. Echocardiography of the aortic root. Invest Radiol 1968; 3:356.

106. Rafferty T, Durkin M. Cardioplegic contrast echocardiography in patients with aortic regurgitation. Anesth Analg 1991; 72:S217.

107. Rafferty T, Durkin M, Elefteriades J, O'Connor T. Transesophageal echocardiographic evaluation of aortic valve integrity using antegrade crystalloid cardioplegia as an imaging agent. J Thorac Cardiovasc Surg (in press).

108. Goldman M, Mindich B, Teichholz L, et al. Intraoperative contrast echocardiography to evaluate mitral valve operations. J Am Coll Cardiol 1984; 4:1035.

109. Goldman M, Fuster V, Guarino T, Mindich B. Intraoperative echocardiography for the evaluation of valvular regurgitation: experience in 263 patients. Circulation 1986; 74:I–143.

110. Lieppe W, Behar V, Schallioni R, Kisslo J. Detection of tricuspid regurgitation with two-dimensional echocardiography and peripheral vein injections. Circulation 1978; 57:128.

111. Goldman M, Mindich B. Intraoperative cardioplegic contrast echocardiography for assessing myocardial perfusion during open heart surgery. J Am Coll Cardiol 1984; 4:1029.

112. Rafferty T, Durkin M, Hines R, O'Connor T. Witnessed right atrial injectate thermodilution right ventricular ejection fraction reproducibility. Anesthesiology 1991; 75:A461.

113. Tei C, Sakamaki T, Shah P, et al. Myocardial contrast echocardiography: a reproducible technique of myocardial opacification for identifying regional perfusion deficits. Circulation 1983; 67:585.

114. Sakamaki T, Tei C, Meerbaum S, et al. Verification of myocardial contrast two-dimensional echocardiographic assessment of perfusion defects in ischemic myocardium. J Am Coll Cardiol 1984; 3:34.

115. Kondo S, Tei C, Meerbaum S, et al. Hyperemic response of intracoronary contrast agents during two dimensional echographic delineation of regional myocardium. J Am Coll Cardiol 1984; 4:49.

116. Kaul S, Pandian N, Okada R, et al. Contrast echocardiography in acute myocardial ischemia. I. In-vivo determination of total left ventricular "area at risk." J Am Coll Cardiol 1984; 4:1272.

117. Gillam L, Kaul S, Fallon J, et al. Functional and pathologic effects of multiple echocardiographic contrast injections on the myocardium, brain and kidneys. J Am Coll Cardiol 1985; 6:687.

118. Kaul S, Gillam L, Weyman A. Contrast echocardiography in acute myocardial ischemia. II. The effect of site of injection of contrast agent on the estimation of area at risk for necrosis after coronary occlusion. J Am Coll Cardiol 1985; 6:825.

119. Armstrong W, Mueller T, Kinney E, et al. Assessment of myocardial perfusion abnormalities with contrast-enhanced two-dimensional echocardiography. Circulation 1982; 66:166.

120. Santoso T, Roelandt J, Mansyoer H, et al. Myocardial perfusion imaging in humans by contrast echocardiography using polygelin colloid solution. J Am Coll Cardiol 1985; 6:612.

121. Berwing K, Schlepper M. Echocardiographic imaging of the left ventricle by peripheral intravenous injection of echo contrast agent. Am Heart J 1988; 115:399.

122. Black S, Muzzi D, Nishimura R, Cucchiara R. Preoperative

and intraoperative echocardiography to detect right to left shunt in patients undergoing neurosurgical procedures in the sitting position. Anesthesiology 1990; 72:436.

123. Keller M, Feinstein S, Briller R, Powsner S. Automated production and analysis of echo contrast agents. J Ultrasound Med 1986; 5:493.

124. Cate T, Drury K, Meerbaum S, et al. Myocardial contrast two-dimensional echocardiography: experimental examination at different coronary flow levels. J Am Coll Cardiol 1984; 3:1219.

125. Feinstein S, Cate T, Zwehl W, et al. Two-dimensional contrast echocardiography. I. In vitro development and quantitative analysis of echo contrast agents. J Am Coll Cardiol 1984; 3:14.

126. Keller M, Glasheen W, Teja K, et al. Myocardial contrast echocardiography without significant hemodynamic effects or reactive hyperemia: a major advantage in the imaging of regional myocardial perfusion. J Am Coll Cardiol 1988; 12:1039.

127. Keller M, Feinstein S, Watson D. Successful left ventricular opacification following peripheral venous injection of sonicated contrast agent: an experimental evaluation. Am Heart J 1987; 114:570.

128. Feinstein S, Shah P, Bing R, et al. Microbubble dynamics visualized in the intact capillary circulation. J Am Coll Cardiol 1984; 4:595.

129. Moore C, Smucker M, Kaul S. Myocardial contrast echocardiography in humans. I. Safety. A comparison with routine coronary arteriography. J Am Coll Cardiol 1986; 8:1066.

130. Cheirif J, Zoghbi W, Raizner A, et al. Assessment of myocardial perfusion in humans by contrast echocardiography. I. Evaluation of regional coronary reserve by peak contrast intensity. J Am Coll Cardiol 1988; 11:735.

131. Spotnitz W, Keller M, Watson D, Nolan S, Kaul S. Success of internal mammary bypass grafting can be assessed intraoperatively using myocardial contrast echocardiography. J Am Coll Cardiol 1988; 12:196.

132. Aronson S, Bender E, Feinstein S, et al. Contrast echocardiography: a method to visualize changes in regional myocardial perfusion in the dog model for CABG surgery. Anesthesiology 1990; 72:295.

133. Akasaka T, Yoshikawa J, Yoshida K, et al. Echocardiographic characteristics and clinical significance of the spontaneous contrast echoes. J Cardiol 1987; 17:159.

134. Castello R, Pearson A, Sobovitz A. Prevalence and clinical implications of atrial spontaneous contrast in patients undergoing transesophageal echocardiography. Am J Cardiol 1990; 65:1149.

135. Pollick C, Taylor D. Assessment of left atrial appendage function by transesophageal echocardiography. Implications for the development of thrombus. Circulation 1991; 84:223.

136. Black I, Hopkins A, Lee L, Walsh W. Left atrial spontaneous echo contrast: A clinical and echocardiographic analysis. J Am Coll Cardiol 1991; 18:398.

137. Chen Y, Kan M, Chen J, et al. Contributing factors to formation of left atrial spontaneous echo contrast in mitral valvular disease. J Ultrasound Med 1990; 9:151.

138. Siegel B, Coelho J, Spigos D, et al. Ultrasonography of blood during statis and coagulation. Invest Radiol 1981; 16:71.

139. Siegel B, Coelho J, Scade S, et al. Effect of plasma proteins and temperature on echogenicity of blood. Invest Radiol 1982; 17:29.

140. Siegel B, Machl J, Bertler J, Justin J. Red cell aggregation as a cause of blood flow echogenicity. Radiology 1983; 148:799.

141. Mahony C, Sublett K, Harrison M. Resolution of spontaneous contrast with platelet disaggregatory therapy (trifluoperazine). Am J Cardiol 1989; 63:1009.

142. Mahony C, Evans J, Spain C. Spontaneous contrast and circulating platelet aggregates. Circulation 1989; 80:II.

143. Meltzer R, Klig V, Visser C, Teicholz L. Spontaneous echocardiographic contrast in the inferior vena cava. Am Heart J 1985; 110:826.

144. Castello R, Pearson A, Fagan L, Labovitz A. Spontaneous echocardiographic contrast in the descending aorta. Am Heart J 1990; 120:915.

145. Evangelista A, Gonzalez T, Garcia-del-Castillo H, et al. Spontaneous echocardiographic contrast in the left ventricle related to aortic insufficiency. Rev Esp Cardiol 1990; 43:581.

146. Doud D, Jacobs W, Moran J, Scanlon P. The natural history of left ventricular spontaneous contrast. J Am Soc Echocardiogr 1990; 3:465.

147. Segal R, Baltazar R, Mower M, Stewart C. Spontaneous contrast visualization of the right side of the heart during echocardiography. Am J Med Sci 1986; 292:363.

148. Mikell F, Asinger R, Elsperger K, Anderson W, Hodges M. Regional status of blood in the dysfunctional left ventricle: echocardiographic detection and differentiation from early thrombosis. Circulation 1982; 66:755.

149. Daniel W, Nellessen U, Schroder E, et al. Left atrial spontaneous contrast in mitral valve disease: an indicator for an increased thromboembolic risk. J Am Coll Cardiol 1988; 11:1204.

150. Rafferty T, Lamantia K, Davis E, et al. Quality assurance in intraoperative transesophageal echocardiography—a critical analysis of a two year experience. J Clin Monitoring 1992; 8:170.

151. Rafferty T: Transesophageal two-dimensional echocardiography in the critically ill: is the Swan-Ganz catheter redundant? Yale J Biol Med 1992; 64:375.

18 Future Applications of Transesophageal Echocardiography

The instrumentation and applications of TEE are changing rapidly (Table 18-1). Currently, the biplane probe with continuous-wave Doppler and the probe with a small caliber shaft for pediatric examination are available. During the next few years, we can expect further miniaturization of the adult TEE probe. The concept of biplane imaging can be expanded to multiplane imaging or wide-field TEE tomography, which would provide a panoramic image of the cardiac and thoracic structures (Figs. 18-1 and 18-2). Volumetric data could then be obtained, making the technique more quantitative. This allows the examiner to better discern structures and their interrelationships in the thorax. Higher-frequency transducers (up to 10 MHz) and the ability to change frequency electronically on the same transducer would permit tissue characterization and visualization and quantitation of coronary artery lesions.

In the operating room, transesophageal imaging is being investigated in conjunction with intracoronary or aortic root injection of various contrast agents, to assess the success of regional myocardial reperfusion postcoronary artery bypass grafting. On-line digital processing and analysis of images using automated edge-detection algorithms will improve quantification of intraoperative myocardial ischemia. In addi-

tion, with simultaneous quad-screen display and digital manipulation of echocardiograms, serial-image evaluation throughout the study will be possible. Alarm systems to warn when wall-motion abnormalities surpass a predesignated normal limit would be helpful for continuous monitoring of left ventricular function.

The availability of temperature sensors, ports through which pacing wires could be introduced, and sensors that can display atrial electrocardiograms are all important aspects of future development. Three-dimensional reconstruction is an exciting development for the future.[2,3] The consistently high quality of three-dimensional TEE images obtained from patients so far is helping its evolution.

Table 18-1. Future Applications of Transesophageal Echocardiography

Smaller probes, 4–6 mm, shorter length
Higher-frequency/multifrequency transducers: 5–10 MHz
Myocardial contrast imaging
Portals for physiologic monitoring
Tissue characterization
Multiplane imaging
Three-dimensional reconstruction of images

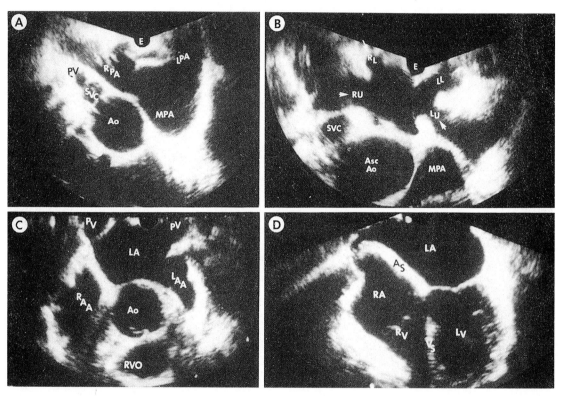

Fig. 18-1. Serial multilevel wide-field transesophageal tomograms, depicting contiguous cardiovascular anatomy. **(A)** Pulmonary arteries and related anatomy. **(B)** Pulmonary veins and related structures. **(C)** Left and right atrial appendages, upper pulmonary veins, and right ventricular outflow tract. **(D)** Dilated cardiac chambers (in different patient). Ao, aorta; AS, atrial septum; Asc Ao, ascending aorta; E, esophagus; LA, left atrium; LAA, left atrial appendage; LL, left lower pulmonary vein; LPA, left pulmonary artery; LU, left upper pulmonary vein; LV, left ventricle; MPA, main pulmonary artery; PV, pulmonary vein; RA, right atrium; RAA, right atrial appendage; RL, right lower pulmonary vein; RPA, right pulmonary artery; RU, right upper pulmonary vein; RV, right ventricle; RVO, right ventricular outflow; SVC, superior vena cava; VS, ventricular septum. (From Seward et al.,[1] with permission.)

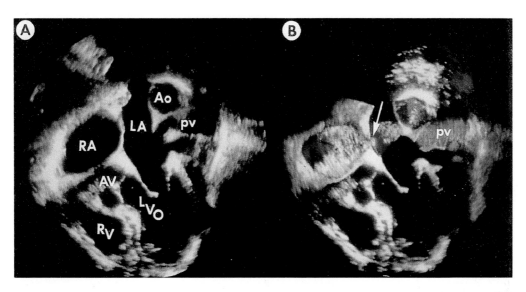

Fig. 18-2. Imaging of cardiothoracic structures in a patient with an atrial septal defect. (A) Wide-field 360-degree tomogram. (B) Color Doppler image demonstrating a left-to-right atrial shunt (arrow). Ao, descending aorta; AV, aortic valve; LA, left atrium; LVO, left ventricular outflow; PV, pulmonary vein; RA, right atrium; RV, right ventricle. (From Seward et al.,[1] with permission.)

REFERENCES

1. Seward JB, Khandheria BK, Tajik AJ. Wide-field transesophageal echocardiographic tomography: feasibility study. Mayo Clin Proc 1990; 65:31–37.
2. Bashein G, Sheehan FH, Nessly ML, et al. 3D transesophageal echo in assessing LV wall motion. J Am Soc Echocardiogr 1991; 4:292 (abst).
3. Hsu TL, Weintraub AR, Ritter SB, Pandian NG. Panoramic transesophageal echocardiography. Echocardiography 1991; 8:677–685.

Index

Page numbers followed by f indicate figures; those followed by t indicate tables.